Praise for *Organic Avenue*

"I discovered Organic Avenue back in 2009, and it has had a profound impact on my relationship with food and the environment. Denise Mari has been an inspiration. This book will make the gap smaller between wanting to do good for yourself and your family and being able to do so. I recommend it highly."

—SENATOR CORY BOOKER

"Denise Mari is a passionate advocate for healthy living—a philosophy that she exposes and lives by. Her simple, powerful vision, embodied in her company, Organic Avenue, changed the nature of the natural-food landscape forever. By combining juicing and a healthy lifestyle, Denise has shown both devoted followers and juicing novices alike how to create health while maintaining a holistic mindful approach to living.

I have recommended Organic Avenue's juices from the very beginning; I consume them myself and continue to advocate their use to my patients as part of a truly healthy lifestyle. Denise Mari is a true pioneer in the field of integrative nutrition and will continue to be a force for many years to come. If you are looking for a way to start a cleanse or are someone who wants to continue on their healthy journey, this is your one must-read book!"

—DR. RICHARD FIRSHEIN, director of the Firshein Center
for Integrative Medicine, author of *The Nutraceutical Revolution,*
The Vitamin Prescription (for Life), and *Reversing Asthma*

"Thank goodness that Denise wanted an *organic* greens juice for herself, then her family, then her friends, and that she wanted it to taste delicious as well as heal the body. Thank goodness that she stood firm—unlike so many before and now after her—on the core principle: '100 percent organic.' Denise trailblazed the path we now all know and rely on: Organic Avenue. And on Organic Avenue she showed the naysayers they were wrong. Yes, you can source, supply, create, and deliver 100 percent organic nutrition in your community, and then to the masses. And yes, you should. I am personally grateful for Denise and her Organic Avenue, and I am professionally grateful for them too."

—ASHLEY KOFF, RD, qualitarian, nutrition expert, author, and speaker

"Organic Avenue has been a great place for me to stop, rejuvenate, and reboot my body and health after all the travel I do for my work. It helps me to keep mentally and spiritually healthy!"

—JESSICA GOMES, actress and model, and six-time
Sports Illustrated Swimsuit Issue model

"Denise Mari is an incredible leader in the juice revolution. Her commitment to spreading awareness about health and wellness is a gift to the world. In her book, *Organic Avenue: Recipes for Life, Made with LOVE*,* she demystifies the process of cleaning your diet and optimizing your health."

—GABRIELLE BERNSTEIN, *New York Times* bestselling author
of *May Cause Miracles*

"If you want to make a difference in this world, you need to start with *you.* This book is your road map to having a rich, healthy life from the inside out. As an ambitious and jet-setting entrepreneur, I adore Organic Avenue and count on the LOVE* lifestyle to keep me fueled and empowered."

—MARIE FORLEO, bestselling author, life coach, and TV personality

"I started a seven-day Organic Avenue juice cleanse, extended it to ten days; after three to four days, I had all of these revelations about how I didn't know the effects of foods that I put in my body. Cleaning myself out with juices, raw soups, and salads changed my experience of and relationship to food."

—TOM SILVERMAN, founder, Tommy Boy Records

"Want to feel fantastic with what you're putting in your precious body? Organic Avenue is my never-fear, go-to beverage whether I'm on the set, traveling, or at home. Thanks to Denise Mari and the Organic Avenue team, I know my body is getting what she deserves. And she loves them all!"

—SHEILA KELLY, founder and CEO, S Factor

"I've been juicing for over a decade and love the way it makes me feel but don't love the preparation. Organic Avenue is awesome because I can buy my juices in advance. They stay fresh, and they taste a lot better than my own!"

—DANIELLE PASHKO, beauty and wellness adviser

"I live in three different countries and travel all over the globe in constant pursuit of the very best nourishment for my body. Denise's nutritious yet delicious creations at Organic Avenue are among the world's finest. They will revitalize and restore your health from the inside out. Her wisdom and vibrant beauty are an excellent testament to how she has mastered the art of wholesome eating."

—RITA THOMAS, LifePilot, philanthropist and health advocate

"Now everyone can get the glow from eating a plant-based, live-food diet that we in New York have been lucky enough to experience through Organic Avenue. It's the only juice-cleanse company I personally use and recommend to my clients. In this book, Denise's vision for a LOVE*-based lifestyle transcends just food, and instead encompasses the entire mind-body-spirit connection, which is the key to ultimate health. A fascinating read that is sure to inspire you to a heightened level of wellness."

—MARIA MARLOWE, CHC, founder of the Bombshell Blueprint

"I used to be forty to fifty pounds overweight about ten years ago, but now I'm finding my balance and most of it has to do with Organic Avenue juices, juices that flood your system with nutrients and vitamins! I walked into Organic Avenue seven years ago and did my first juice cleanse—let's be honest—to drop weight quickly, but that cleanse led me to meet so many amazing people and buy my first juicer."

—TRACY JAI EDWARDS, actress, singer, dancer

organic avenue

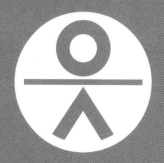

*Live. Organic. Vegan. Experience.

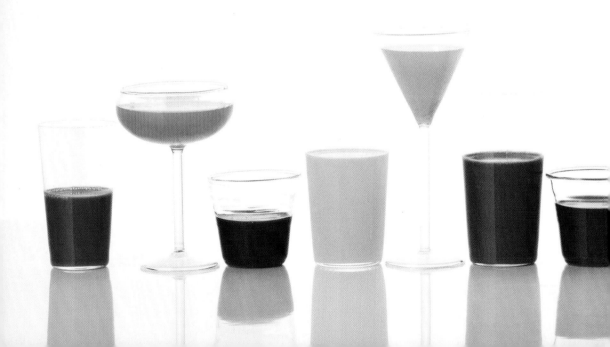

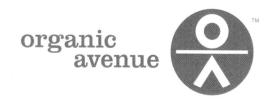

organic
avenue

Recipes for Life,
Made with LOVE*

Denise Mari
with Leda Scheintaub

CONTRIBUTING WRITER Debra Winter
PHOTOGRAPHY BY Quentin Bacon
RECIPE CREATIVE DIRECTION AND STYLING BY ABC Carpet & Home

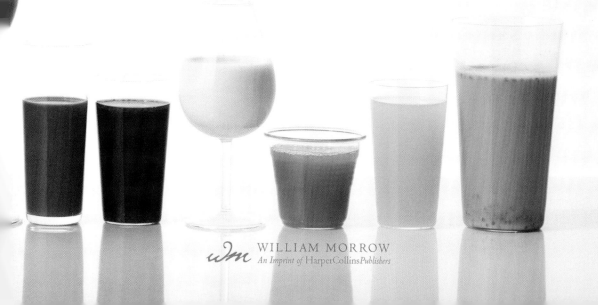

WILLIAM MORROW
An Imprint of HarperCollinsPublishers

This book contains advice and information relating to health care. It is not intended to replace medical advice and should be used to supplement rather than replace regular care by your doctor. It is recommended that you seek your physician's advice before embarking on any medical program or treatment. All efforts have been made to assure the accuracy of the information contained in this book as of the date of publication. The publisher and the author disclaim liability for any medical outcomes that may occur as a result of applying the methods suggested in this book.

HarperCollins books may be purchased for educational, business, or sales promotional use. For information please e-mail the Special Markets Department at SPsales@harpercollins.com.

FIRST EDITION

Library of Congress Cataloging-in-Publication Data has been applied for.

ISBN 978-0-06-220221-5

14 15 16 17 18 OV/RRD 10 9 8 7 6 5 4 3 2 1

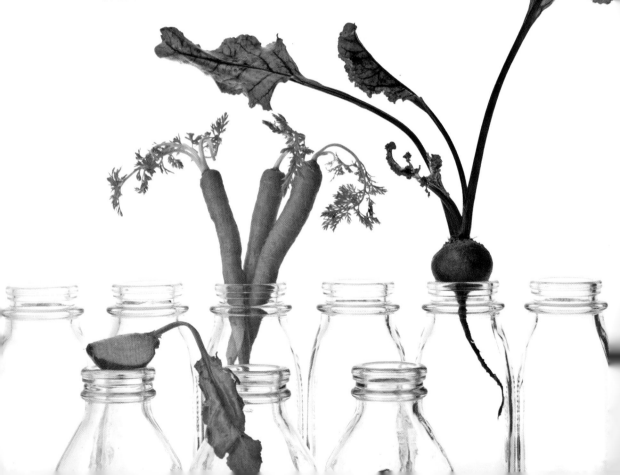

To the sweet guiding light of my sister Kimberly, and the energy of sacrifice and unconditional love of my mom, Dorothy. Their early passings sparked in me purpose and passion, and the ability to realize the precious gifts I have been given: life and love."

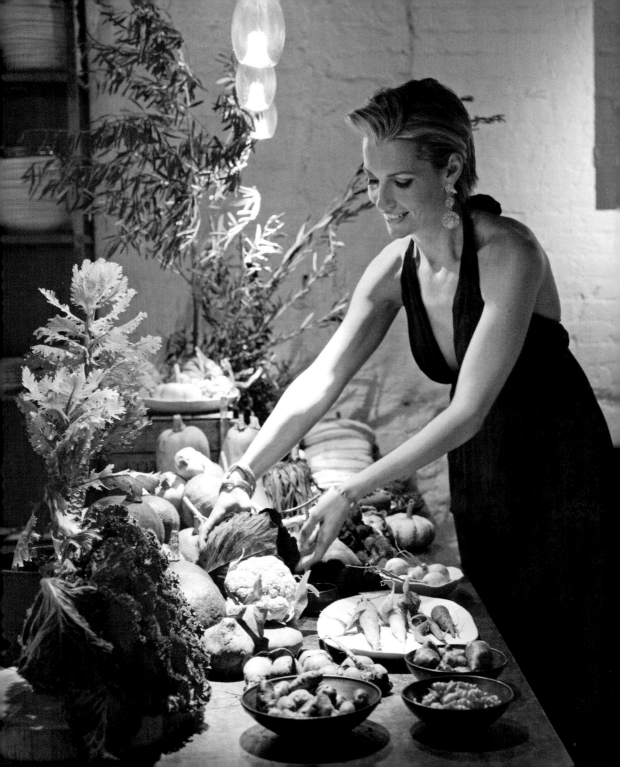

Contents

Foreword

I was raised eating meat just like most other Americans. I believed that finishing my dinner and gulping down my milk would make me grow up to be big and strong. I was given a familiar message that kids (and parents!) are still being spoon-fed today. Never once did I consider exactly what I was eating or what had happened to the animal before it reached my plate. I did have my vegan friends around me, such as my assistant, Simone Reyes, and my good friend Glen E. Friedman, always pounding me with reasons to join their team, but it wasn't until about fifteen years ago when I began taking yoga classes at the Jivamukti Yoga center in New York City that I became vegetarian. I credit the teachings at that school with many life-altering changes: a newfound respect for my body, quieting my mind through meditation, and transforming my eating habits. Up until that time, a hamburger was something stuck between two buns, not a cow; a wing was something you dipped in BBQ sauce, not a chicken; and milk was something you drank as a human, never realizing it was only meant for a calf.

Yoga continues to teach me many things; perhaps most important is the concept of nonviolence in *every* aspect of my life as a global citizen of the world. The more I opened myself up to the idea of the full scope of exactly what nonviolence translates to, the less interested I became in consuming the energy associated with the flesh of an animal that only knew suffering in its life and pain and terror in its death. The more I learned about factory farming and the cruelty animals raised for food must endure before they are led (or dragged) to slaughter, the more I realized that I could not, in good conscience, be a contributor to such violence.

Denise Mari and Organic Avenue represent this type of compassionate living. Organic Avenue has made the vegan lifestyle more accessible, and it is one of the few food and juice companies I trust. I love the convenience of waking up and having my fridge filled with juice and raw food. Now, with this book, Denise shares her vision with the whole country, not just the few who happen to live in New York.

—Russell Simmons

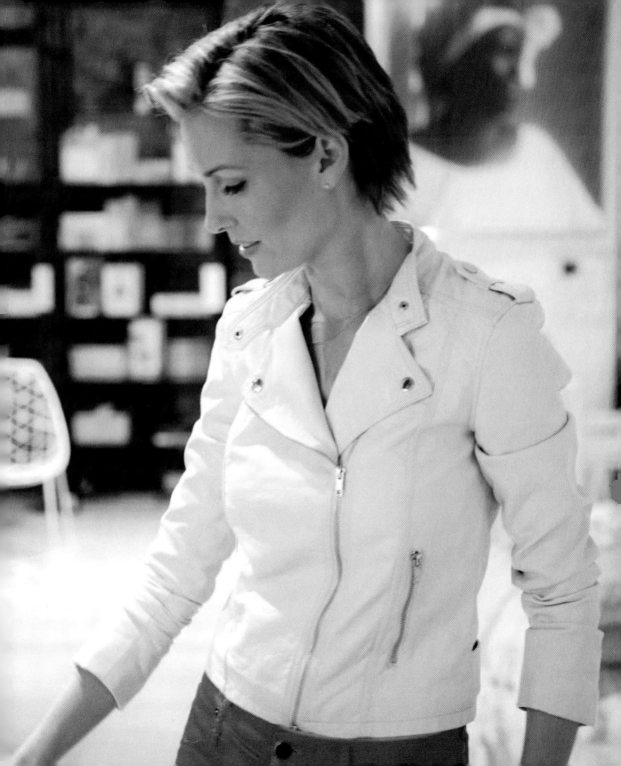

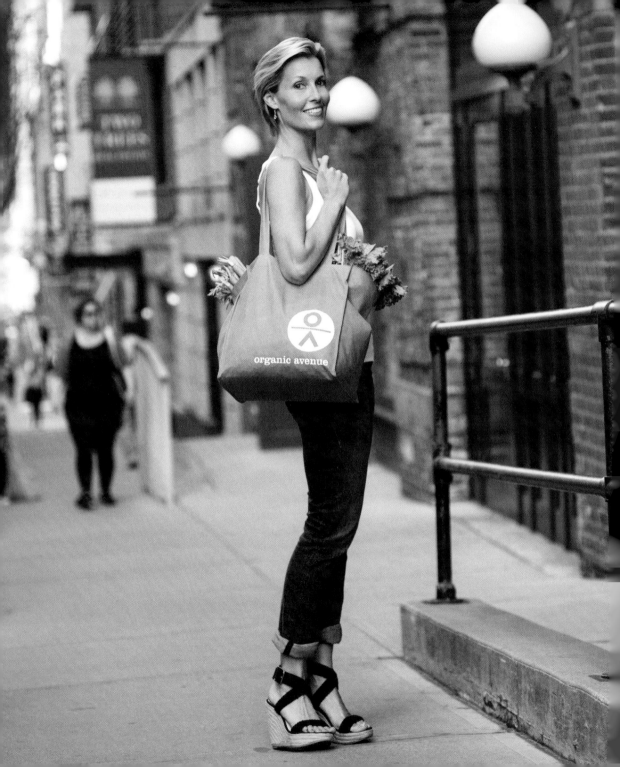

Preface: Why LOVE*? The Organic Avenue Experience

The concept of LOVE* has its roots in my life's journey, beginning with an early attraction to *ahimsa*, or nonviolent consciousness. Ahimsa inspired me to do no harm to the animals, the planet, or myself by following the path of veganism, and to share what I had learned along the way with as many people as possible. The seed for Organic Avenue was planted early, a dream that has turned into a multimillion-dollar business dedicated to supporting others, whether they're dabbling with a cleanse, upgrading current eating habits, or going deeper into a vegetarian and/or vegan living foods lifestyle.

I felt the best way to share and inspire others was to create Organic Avenue retail environments that encouraged a sense of community around the lifestyle. I've always referred to the Organic Avenue retail stores as boutiques. The feeling I wanted to share was clean and simple yet also exciting. The in-store experience was to be the opposite of how natural food stores are often perceived: Rather than with messy bulk bins, dusty shelves, and old wooden floorboards, I'd show-case a chic vegan lifestyle with modern décor, minimal walls, bamboo floors, and a rainbow of bold colors radiating from the iconic milkman-style juice-filled jars.

Yet even more important than the aesthetic of the boutiques, I made it a point to find passionate, knowledgeable staff who complemented our grow-ing community of health-, earth-, and animal-conscious individuals. I wanted people to learn, feel comfortable asking questions, and leave confident they'd found the best product for them—in fact, the best product available! I wanted the boutiques to be part of a full circle of professionals dedicated to making the world a better place, one person at a time.

As the orange and white Organic Avenue logo began to appear with greater regularity on New York City sidewalks, a celebrity following developed. Our bright orange tote bags are now seen throughout the city, a reflection of a growing attraction to LOVE*: the Live. Organic. Vegan. Experience.

Our innovative LOVE*Cleanse programs featuring organic juices, tonics, mylks, and live foods are the foundation of all offerings at Organic Avenue. Yet Organic Avenue is more than just cleansing; it's about the whole experience, and now, with this book, we bring that experience home.

This book will first take you through the letters of LOVE*, spelling out just what goes into the Live. Organic. Vegan. Experience., the backbone of Organic Avenue and a reflection of my health and wellness mission. Then I will introduce you to the world of the LOVE*Cleanse with four different customizable cleanse options: LOVE*Easy, LOVE*Fast, LOVE*Deep, and Go Green. I will go into detail about each and help you decide which is best for you. I will hold your hand and share with you everything I've learned about cleansing over the years: the reasons we should cleanse, how to start out, what to expect along the way, and how to transition back to eating—creating a new normal based on nutritious, mouthwatering food that is 100 percent cruelty-free. Then I will jump-start your entry into Organic Avenue living with a treasure trove of recipes, including a large selection of juices, smoothies, salads, soups, wraps and other main dishes, and desserts to tempt your taste buds.

Cleansing is more than just a hot new trend; it is a healthy lifestyle tool for the ages, and cleansing the Organic Avenue way is practical, sustainable, and infinitely doable. Pounds lost, health regained, and off-the-charts energy are strong motivators, and it is my sincere hope that with this book you will be inspired to stay the course. **Do it for the LOVE* of it!**

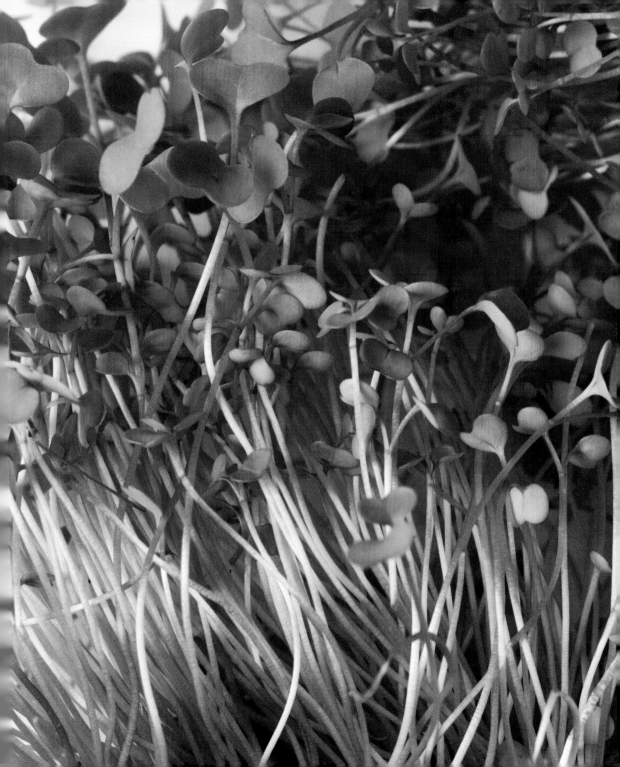

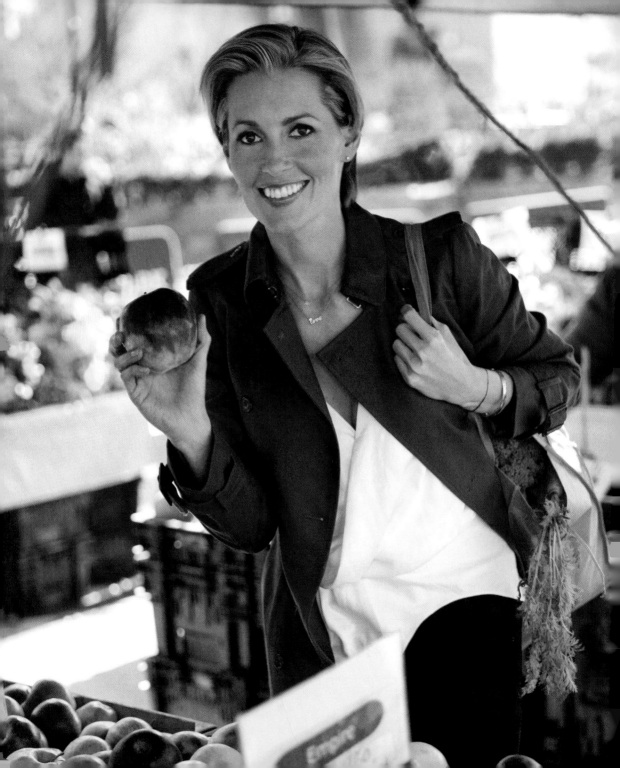

Introduction

Denise Mari and the Spark That Ignited Organic Avenue

People often ask me how I came to create Organic Avenue. I pause, take a deep breath, then sincerely reach to a place deep in my heart and remember when the original spark was ignited. I appreciate the whole of my past experience, the bright and dark days of my early childhood, the highs and lows, the excitement and loss, the willpower and faith, all of which created the parameters of the life I have lived. It's my greatest wish that reading my story will inspire positive change, as my journey has showed me how to turn losing into living.

As I mentioned earlier, the Organic Avenue journey all began with an ahimsa consciousness, a concept known here in the West by our exposure to the great teachings of Mahatma Gandhi. In Sanskrit, *ahimsa* literally means "to do no harm" and is an important tenet in many religions, including Buddhism, Hinduism, and Jainism. Ahimsa encourages embracing a nonviolent way of living. Similarly, as a child I was exposed to a Christian upbringing, so my earliest influence was outlined in biblical terms with the commandment "Thou shalt not kill." Later I came to hear of a great prophet named Mohammed who was quoted as saying, "Whoever is kind to the creatures of God is kind to himself." Eventually I came to understand that from Abraham and Moses and before, and transcending religion, culture, class, and country, you'll find many a guidepost pointing us toward a peaceful way of living.

❝ *In a gentle way, you can shake the world."*

—MAHATMA GANDHI

As I experienced life, loss, and love, I realized the need for purposeful action, to make meaningful contributions with my time and energy. My hopes were that along the journey I could help others who needed some encouragement, an example to follow, or simply recipes for life.

I realized that many people did not have access to the life-changing information, the education, the healthful food and fresh organic juice, and the supportive community needed to embrace this type of positive life change. I didn't always have it either! Little did I know that my journey was delivering me toward realizing my greatest aspirations. I developed the concept of Organic Avenue from a daydreamlike vision to a multimillion-dollar enterprise serving the one thing I cared most about, and something I truly wanted to contribute in this lifetime: LOVE*. Organic Avenue would come to embody this LOVE*, the acronym standing for the Live. Organic. Vegan. Experience., a business dedicated to encouraging others to do better for one other, the animals, and the planet.

Once upon a Lifetime

They say everything happens for a reason. In many ways, I believe this to be true. However, when it came to losing my little sister to cancer, the "reason" was less than clear and the importance of honoring life became the lesson.

We were a seemingly healthy family of six: my parents; my sisters, Kimberly and Michele; my brother, John; and me. We'd never heard of the term *organic*, and we didn't know anyone who claimed to be a vegetarian. In other words, it was the basic American lifestyle. It all seemed normal at the time, but looking back on it now, I can see the role it may have played in my family's health. We enjoyed everything the typical American family of the time enjoyed, from Happy Meals to TV dinners. The standard American diet (now known as "SAD") was all we knew. Hamburgers, pizza, mac and cheese, soda, white rice, vegetables from a can, cooked meat, and pasteurized milk. At that time the addictive effects of many ingredients in these foods, such as high-fructose corn syrup, and allergies to wheat and dairy were not common knowledge. In fact, there was a time fructose was looked upon as a fruit-based sweetener and considered a healthier option. Then there was sugar on everything. If you had a grapefruit, you'd put sugar on it. If you had sugared cereal, you'd put sugar on it. We ate very little unprocessed food, and iceberg lettuce was about as raw as things got on our dinner table.

A shock hit my family's reality when after a yearlong battle involving hospitals, chemo, and heartbreak, we lost Kimberly to cancer. She was two years younger than me, and through her passing, I sensed my mortality for the first time. As I looked at her in the open coffin, I tried to grasp the whole meaning of this tragedy, but at eight years old my heart simply swelled with a grief that I could not fully process. We all did our best to pick up the pieces and carry on, but I was forever changed. If it had happened to her, it could happen to us—any of us. A heavy weight for any mother, father, or child to bear. Yet this life journey ultimately spares no one, and the sooner we realize this, the sooner we can make greater use of all our moments. For me that realization was to have a direct influence on my life choices, leading to my explorations into vegetarianism, veganism, and raw foodism, and, ultimately, to the birth of Organic Avenue.

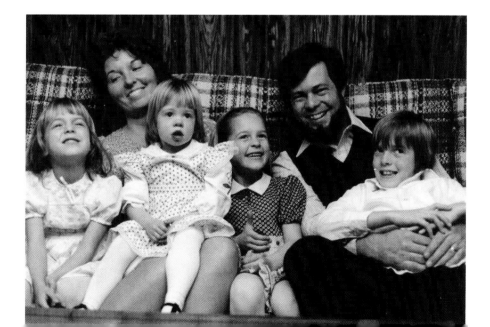

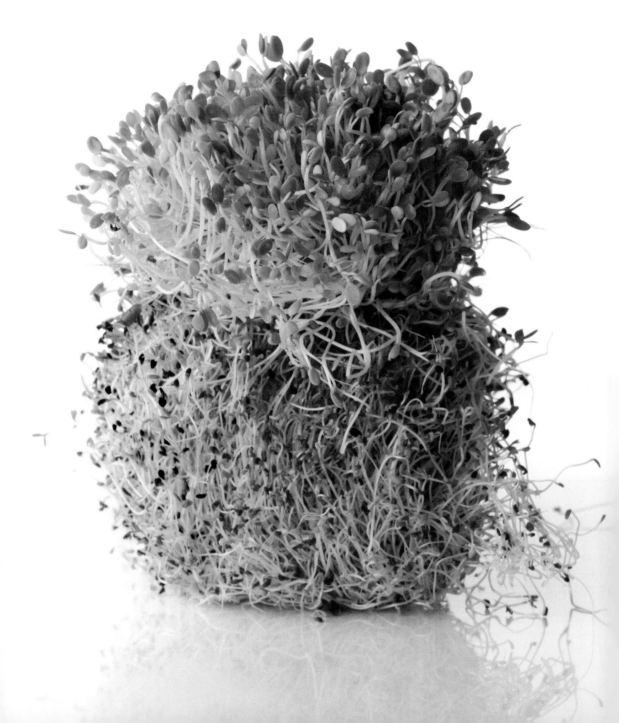

Flirting with Vegetarianism

❝ I cannot fish without falling a little in self-respect."
—HENRY DAVID THOREAU

I always loved animals, but it wasn't until a fishing trip with my dad that I connected my love of animals with becoming a vegetarian. It was a perfect day. I caught a fish. But clarity came at the moment my father began to prepare the grill and the fish was lying on the table. At that moment something clicked inside. I was never going to eat fish again. I couldn't.

❝ I did not become a vegetarian for my health, I did it for the health of the chickens."
—ISAAC BASHEVIS SINGER

At first I became an **ovo-lacto vegetarian**, a type of vegetarian who eats no animal flesh but does consume eggs and animal by-products. Milk, cheese, eggs, and butter were still on the menu. I continued to educate myself, asked deeper questions, and learned to read labels. My friends and family would often comment that it was a multihour episode just to go grocery shopping with me. I found that meat by-products were in the weirdest places: Cheese is regularly made with rennet (from the stomach of animals), meaning many cheeses aren't truly vegetarian, and common table sugar is often refined with animal bones. I learned a whole new way to navigate and select the foods that I felt were good for me—and the animals. I wanted to share my new devotion to this ideology that supported my growing belief that what I consumed mattered and that what I chose had a life-or-death consequence for another innocent being. I felt responsible. I took it upon myself to find out the truth behind the food and animal industry. The deeper I looked for answers, the more I was astounded, even

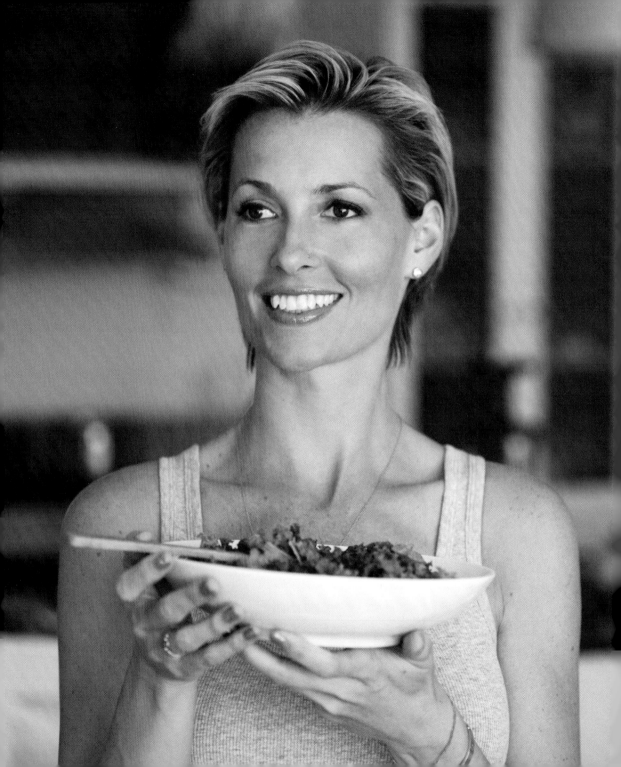

scared! I discovered that torture was the effect of the choice of eating meat and environmental destruction was the consequence of raising the animals for food, and to me it didn't add up. The more I looked, the more I learned, and the more I was encouraged by the promise of a plant-based diet. I felt the direct link between my food and where it came from; the implications it had on my health, my energy level, and my physical being; and the impact it had on the animals and the environment. I needed to lighten my impact. I needed to take responsibility for my actions. One step at a time.

VISION OF LOVE: JUST ONE OTHER PERSON

Gandhi said, "Be the change you wish to see in the world," and that particularly resonated with me. When I first became a vegetarian, I had a clear but powerful insight: If I could influence just one other person to become vegetarian, then my life would have meaning. And I didn't have to teach or preach—I merely had to learn and be. It was I who had to lead the change by being the change and then I would witness the change around me. It felt awesome to have this connection and knowledge.

The Love Goes Deeper: Vegan Awakening

As I learned more about the destructive and animal-abusive practices that yielded some vegetarian foods (milk, cheese, eggs), I became intrigued by the concept of **veganism:** eating no animal products, including eggs and dairy. I wanted to see these "vegans": Who were they? What did they look like? Did they look healthy? Were they truly able to keep up a healthy diet? Could I become a vegan and still indulge? What would I have to give up? What new foods would I be adding? Did I need to add supplements? Could I do it?

As I began to meet real live vegans, I would come to understand veganism as a truly commonsense approach to eating. Once I committed to the vegan lifestyle, a whole new world opened up. I felt better and looked better. I lost weight, my skin cleared up, and my clarity of mind and purpose resonated loudly. It was easier than I thought!

Another aspect of veganism is raw foodism, an integral part of the LOVE*Lifestyle and the backbone of this book. Some commit to it 100 percent and others in intervals for the purpose of cleansing. A truly healthy vegan eats an abundance of raw plant-based foods. As I researched the benefits of eating solely raw foods—fruits, vegetables, nuts, seeds, seaweeds, sprouts, and grasses in their raw, unheated state with very limited processing—it all made sense to me. I decided to try it myself.

VISION OF LOVE: BEING THE CHANGE

People were seeing something changing in me. One day I heard a voice inside me say, "It's about being and attracting." At the time, I was meeting new and inspired people; I studied everything I could get my hands on, attended health lectures and worked for the gurus of the moment, took cutting-edge courses that offered information that conventional schools weren't talking about, about everything from colonics to counseling, and topped it all off with a mini education in entrepreneurship (thanks to my dear friend and soon-to-be business partner, Doug Evans). I knew that the lifestyle (not just the diet) had to be made convenient, delicious, accessible, affordable, and most of all fun. Little did I know I was well on my way to becoming a vegan, and Organic Avenue was well on its way to having a business plan.

*** *Being vegan helped me realize I can say and do what I believe is right. That's powerful."*

—ALICIA SILVERSTONE

Going Raw: Deepening the Dedication

Raw foods were truly transformative: Could this be as good as it seemed? I was hearing so many apparently miraculous reports of people's illnesses reversing course, and people I knew were consistently experiencing radiant, glowing good health on a raw foods diet. It was an inspiring time!

The early days were filled with euphoria and clarity as I inundated my body with organic green juices and raw fruits and vegetables. The most exciting part of this initial cleansing journey was the feeling that I had a clear purpose and motivation, coupled with the energy needed to take action.

My goal here on earth was becoming clearer. I had a vision of Organic Avenue as a place where people could find everything they needed either to maintain a high-raw, whole-foods, plant-based vegan diet and lifestyle or to integrate whatever parts of the lifestyle matched the path they were currently on, be it vegetarianism or a simple upgrade to their eating patterns. I wanted to offer people a foundation of products and services that would save time and reduce the feeling of deprivation associated with the "giving up" aspect of the journey. I was getting a glimpse of my ultimate purpose: the launching of Organic Avenue.

[xxix]

*** *When you know you need to change, there are two ways to do it: struggle and suffer or just surrender. Surrender is* **soooo** *much easier. Just visualize letting go . . . feel the loss of power the object, person, or food has on you . . . and be amazed at how all of a sudden* **you can** *rather than* **you can't.** *"*

—DENISE MARI

Beginning to Share the LOVE*

My passion for the LOVE*Lifestyle was intensifying, and I was ready to share it with others. I literally set up shop in my second-floor apartment on New York City's Lower East Side: I brought in all types of raw food staples, superfoods, and supplements, and I launched the Organic Avenue LOVE*Cleanse, the first NYC-based juicing and cleansing program. With all my credit cards maxed, and with supportive friends, a niche community to serve, and fingers crossed, I threw myself completely into my life's passion. At that time, cleanses were something people left New York City to do. They often were for the elite, very ill, or addicted, and they were *expensive.* I thought, Why not begin to offer cleanses right here? Why not deliver them right from my home? I was on a mission, and my naïveté paid off. I wanted everyone to be able to experience the lifestyle, and I knew that the more people experienced it, the more they would love it. Just as the cleansing and inundation of high-quality nutrition was what was sparking my clarity and intense devotion, I thought if others had the opportunity to cleanse, then they, too, would have their own personal revelations. It could only mean more good on the planet.

If I had known then what I know now, I probably never would have started my business. I had no idea what kind of logistic nightmare the delivery of fresh juice and food could be in the metropolis of Manhattan. The force toward building Organic Avenue was becoming irrepressible: I'd work out the logistics. I was determined to make this lifestyle available to more people. My feet were on the ground, and the only way I could go was up!

The Boom of Organic Avenue and LOVE*: Passion with Purpose

My passion was overflowing, yet doing business from my Lower East Side apartment had its challenges; eventually my neighbors in the apartment above me started to complain about the sound of the juicer and blender going at three in the morning. So after a few years of running a truly home-based operation, I was excited to move into my first retail space. With a few extra hands, we were fast and furiously making juice, raw food, and LOVE*Cleanse packages and delivering them around the city using any form of transportation available, from bicycle messengers to car services! I did a lot of everything, from working the register to creating the marketing materials, ordering the products, stocking the shelves, and, of course, making the juice. I knew little about business, but I had a clear vision in mind and was firm in my resolve to make it happen.

The business was growing fast, and I was well on the way to realizing my heart and soul's mission: to create a better world by helping people, animals, and the environment. My first business partner, Doug Evans, worked away at a high-tech job and helped infuse seed money into this budding business. Every ounce of energy was needed to prove that this vision was far more than a hobby, that what I was doing was laying the foundation for the global enterprise I knew Organic Avenue could become.

My motto became "Do It for the LOVE* of It!" And though it was not easy, it truly was a labor of love.

[xxxi]

❝ *Live an intentional life."*

—DENISE MARI

Organic Avenue Growing Up: Spreading the LOVE*

Soon the Organic Avenue kitchen was starting to burst at the seams. We decided that if we wanted to make the business work on a large scale, we would need to take on a larger kitchen facility with expansion capabilities. From here it became a race: The business was expanding exponentially and people were loving the products; other entrepreneurs also loved the idea, and new competition was brewing in the city. We had first mover advantage, and the city became decorated with our bright orange reusable and recyclable bags. Almost everyone seemed to know of Organic Avenue. Good things were being said. People were taking the LOVE*Cleanse challenge and were reporting great results. They would recommend it to their friends. Groups started signing up for cleanses. Celebrities led the way and paparazzi shot pictures of them on the streets of New York and on music sets—wherever you looked, there were the orange bags or iconic bottles. My partner and I lived the lifestyle and enthusiastically shared our experiences whenever we could. Life was good!

Loving, Learning, and Letting Go

I was living my dream until one day I received a call that would again change my life forever. It was from my dad. He asked if I was sitting down: My mother had been diagnosed with cancer. My mother, beautiful soul, was given the same news as my sister Kimberly. Instead of a happy retirement, my parents were to relive the experience of hospitals, chemo, and all that goes along with conventional cancer treatment. Within a year, I lost my mom.

Through the despair I could see that the Universe throws us experiences for greater learning and inquiry. I reflected on the past. By the time I reached college I had counted too many funerals. I experienced the loss of Kimberly to cancer, one grandfather to stroke, the other grandfather to emphysema, and a grandmother to complications of type 2 diabetes. My brother had a brain tumor removed successfully, and my father is surviving cancer that required surgical intervention. And now I added my mother to the list, lost to cancer. As I was learning about the promise of prevention and alternative treatments for cancer and other serious illnesses, I looked back in time and wondered whether some of this could have been prevented. With that lingering question, loving and letting go became my next life lesson.

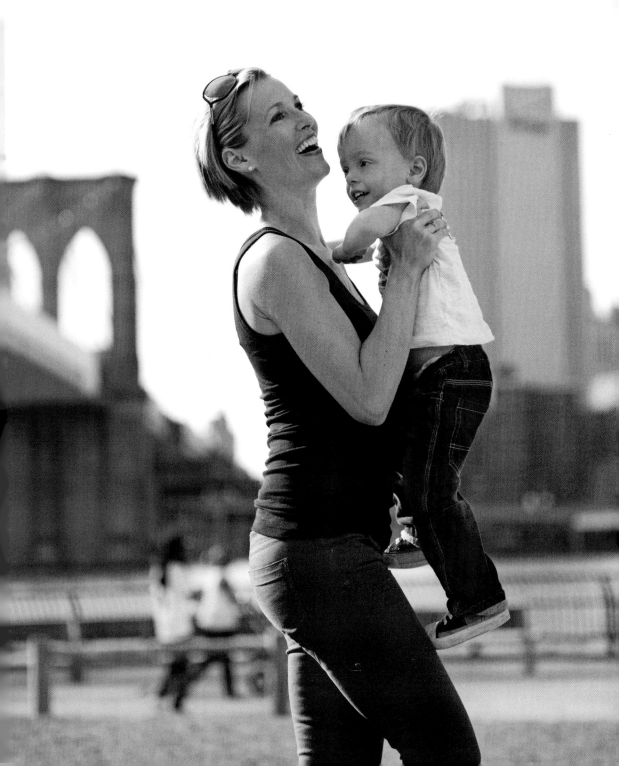

❝ I will greet this day with love in my heart."

—OG MANDINO

Mission Possible: Bring on the LOVE*!

We are given no specific guidebook on how to live. Each person is met with a unique situation. Our immediate examples can often be both inspiring and detrimental. We are born into our circumstances, and until we can master our realities and change those circumstances, life has its way with us. Life itself takes us on a journey; our emotions, reactions, and experiences mold and shape us. Sometimes the dark, deep despair and the loneliness and loss of loved ones shape us most.

My journey brought me to a place where I feel full of faith in the magical and mystical, as well as grateful for the traditional wisdom that points toward a compassionate and joy-filled existence. Even in the knowledge of mortality there is still a sense of promise of the immortal, both here on earth by right living and in the afterlife according to eternal guidelines. I believe that Organic Avenue and the LOVE*Lifestyle offer hope and the tools to begin, all the while providing support along the way. Each of us will suffer bumps and bruises as we move along our individual paths, and not all answers will come to us immediately. We all have different health and lifestyle goals, be it to lose weight, ease a health condition, or support an already dedicated vegan lifestyle. You may relate directly to my story, maybe to part of it; wherever you are is your unique place on the journey in your life. Yet you can be promised that as you fill your body with the juices and food shared in the chapters to follow, you, too, will have an awakening, a powerful insight, new energy, motivation, and, God willing, a passionate and purposeful life to follow. In the spirit of love, I offer you the complete experience, recipes for life, made with LOVE*.

organic avenue

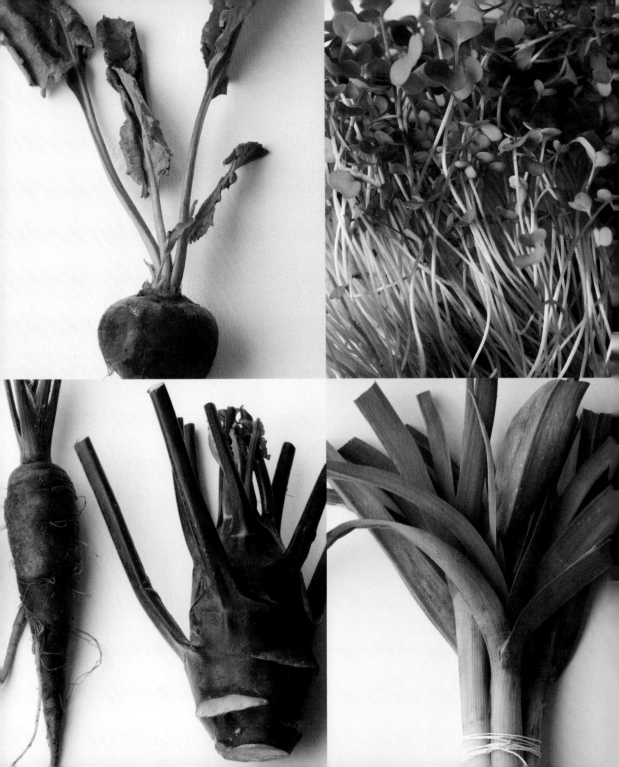

PART I

What Is LOVE*?

LOVE* is the founding and guiding principle of Organic Avenue. LOVE* is the manifestation of my life's purpose, starting from my earliest vegetarian inclinations to my embrace of the living foods lifestyle, and it became my motto many years ago as a way to keep my dietary choices and business goals aligned with my greatest mission. Breaking down the acronym into its four components—the Live. Organic. Vegan. Experience.—gives us guidance on how we can eat and live in the most health-promoting, environmentally pure, and animal-friendly way possible. How do you bring LOVE* into all you do and are? Start with the food you eat and work your way out from there. After all, what you put into your body says a lot about who you are; as the old saying goes, you are what you eat!

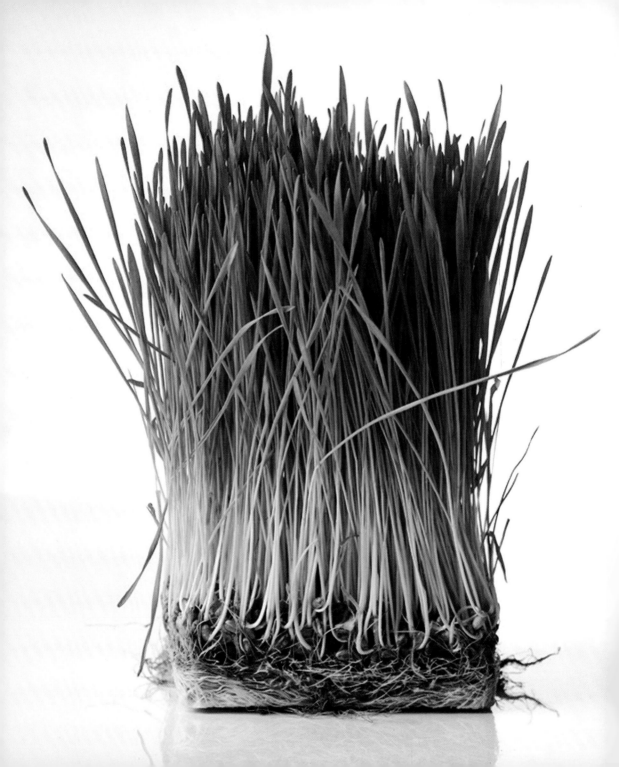

LOVE*: THE LIVE. ORGANIC. VEGAN. EXPERIENCE.

Live: Plant-based, enzymatically active, energetically alive foods

Organic: Nutrient-rich, pure, non-GMO, organically grown foods

Vegan: Ahimsa (nonviolent), compassionate way of living, animal friendly

Experience: Lifestyle, holistic practice, and the sum of incorporating all the elements of LOVE*

LOVE*: A Quick Overview

Many of us familiar with Organic Avenue think of LOVE* as synonymous with our signature cleanses. Yes, our cleanses incorporating fresh juices, smoothies, nut mylks, and living foods have developed quite a following, but LOVE* is also about the bigger lifestyle picture. This section of the book introduces us to the core concepts of LOVE*, the *what* and *why* of living plant-based foods, the importance of going organic, and an introduction to daily lifestyle practices. In short:

[3]

- **L** is for live foods (also known as raw foods), those in their pure, unheated state with their most vibrant, alive properties intact. I believe that the earth has provided all the living foods—fruits, vegetables, grains, legumes, nuts, seeds, and seaweeds—that humans need to thrive. Taking the emphasis off the animal kingdom for human foods allows the LOVE* concept to count for *all* sentient beings.
- **O** is for organic; the more you understand how deeply pollution, pesticides, poisoning, and genetic modification affect the food we eat, the more organic becomes a goal. Organic Avenue goes a step further than organic, not simply adhering to the official definition of the word but also ensuring that we're getting the very best on the market by favoring suppliers who use the most sustainable practices.

- **V** is for vegan. This means plant-based and extends beyond food to clothing and other consumables. I once saw Jane Goodall speak and was motivated by her dedication to animal rights and a vegetarian diet. Her philosophy—"What you do makes a difference, and you have to decide what kind of difference you want to make"—says it all to me. For me, making a difference means following a nonviolent, LOVE* lifestyle.
- **E** is for experience, connecting the elements of LOVE* to capture big-picture clarity: finding connection with those on a similar path, meditating to mend the mind, exercising to further support a healthy lifestyle, and continuing to live, love, and let go.

LOVE + LOVE*

What could be better than to look at love both as a principle to live by and as the central theme of the food you eat? I find solace in knowing that promoting the LOVE*Lifestyle is contributing to greater peace, health, and happiness both on the planet and within myself, and I'm certain that you will feel the same too. Yes, we play with an acronym, but don't let it fool you. We are focused on the larger meaning of the word *love,* and our wish is to help provide the tools for you to easily adopt this peaceful way of life. It is a rewarding way to live. Striving to be that positive change gives us a unique opportunity to control our destiny, to use our power of choice, to live and thrive in a way that is, quite simply, not harmful. Not to be perfect, but to work to improve every step of the way.

Those eager to jump in can skip directly to the LOVE*Cleanse section (pages 39 to 105), but first familiarizing yourself with the concepts of LOVE* will give you a firm foundation with which to make the smartest choices. Depending on where you are and where you want to go, you can incorporate some or all of LOVE* into your life: You can dive right in with a juice cleanse, simply green up your diet a bit, or take the plunge and become a vegetarian, a vegan, or a raw foodie! Find what speaks to you: Baby steps and large lifestyle shifts are equally welcome! In the subsequent sections, I'll introduce the LOVE*Cleanses, followed by the Organic Avenue recipes, giving you the tools to implement a LOVE*-based diet and thus affect the changes that we tempt you with here.

The emphasis is not to see how much you can give up. On the contrary, it's about enjoying a healthy, love-filled life that includes delicious foods. Organic Avenue will help you to establish a new normal: an everyday diet based on LOVE* principles that are practical, sustainable, and doable.

Time to go through the letters one by one and invite you into the space of LOVE*.

❝ *Love and compassion are necessities, not luxuries. Without them humanity cannot survive."*

—DALAI LAMA

[5]

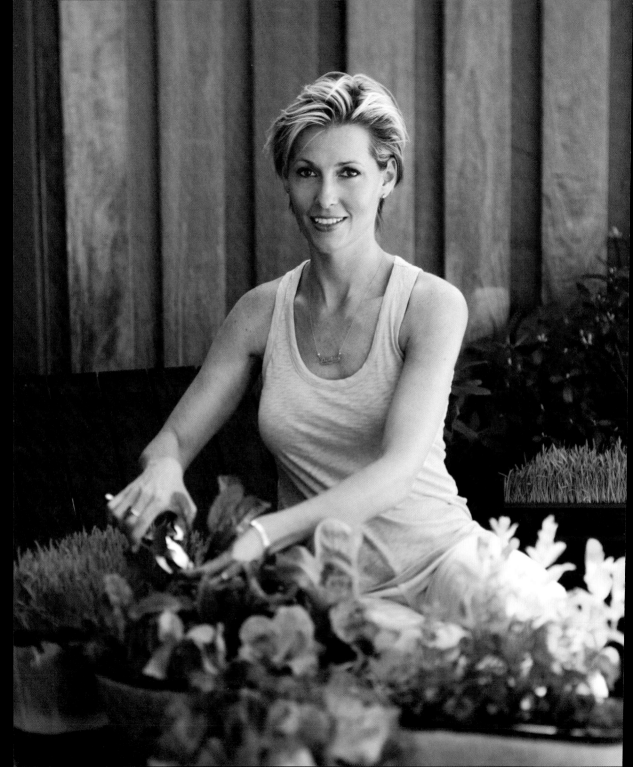

L = Live (Līv)

Live foods are synonymous with raw foods. At Organic Avenue, we strive to eat 80 percent raw, enzymatically alive, organic foods (we'll get into definitions below) and 20 percent wholesome plant-based organic consciously cooked foods. *Plant-based* is the key, as a plant-based diet is at the very core of LOVE*. While most plant-based foods can be consumed raw or cooked, we have found that the more raw food we eat, the higher level of health we experience. And when we're experiencing illness, eating 100 percent raw foods or juicing for a period of time allows the bodily systems to do what they do best without the diversion and energetic drain of digesting cooked foods.

Is Raw Radical or Rational?

What did you have for lunch? If your answer is "a salad," you are one third of the way to a life with more energy, vitality, and health! You are intuitively heading in the direction of LOVE*. If your answer is not remotely close to that salad and you are struggling with a symptom or stubborn excess weight, then be very excited. We've got a solution that you will enjoy and see results from right away.

Let's turn mainstream reasoning on its head for a moment: I'd like to suggest that *cooking* is a lot more radical than eating raw, or "live," as I like to refer to this vitality-promoting way of eating. If vibrancy had a color, what would it be? Green, of course, the color of that salad. Let's say it's a spinach salad. Now take that spinach and picture it at the other extreme: canned. Cooked at a super-high temperature with a shelf life of years rather than days. But at the cost of life, literally: Canned foods are considered good to go when they are *sterile,* which means "free from living organisms"!

If "Why raw?" is your question, then "Heat hurts" is my answer. Although some will find an argument against this simple natural law (yes, those cooked tomatoes and their heightened lycopene content did create quite a stir), others can intuitively understand that unadulterated raw foods (think apples, lettuce greens, carrots) have living enzymes (energy catalysts), intact amino acids (building blocks of protein), vitamins, minerals, and a host of macro- and micronutrients. This is what is attracting more and more people to the foods of LOVE*.

A general temperature guideline is a 118-degree heat limit for keeping foods live; above this temperature things change. Although we like to think all change is for the good, it's not always the case: When food is heated, the change in chemical composition is not so good. Vitamins are destroyed, enzymes are inactivated, and proteins are denatured. It's a hot mess! And if you are boiling your veggies, you are pouring out an abundance of minerals along with that water.

DID YOU KNOW?

The science of canning came about not as an advance in food nutrition but as to way to ward off sheer starvation during the Napoleonic Wars. After enemy armies burned fields and food as they retreated, canned food was a lifesaver. Sure, canned food will keep you alive, but living foods will keep you living to the fullest. And who wants to be minimally alive when you can thrive?

Living foods help restore harmony in the body. They nourish, cleanse, and alkalize the body. Living foods are high in vitamins, minerals, amino acids, complex carbohydrates, fiber, oxygen, and enzymes. Some experts believe the human body is designed to live beyond one hundred years, and that a "raw," "live," or LOVE*Lifestyle and diet make that a real possibility.

To pique your interest, here's a partial list of whole foods beginning with the letter *a.* Imagine what the rest of the alphabet will bring! (Take a look at Rebecca Wood's *New Whole Foods Encyclopedia* for a comprehensive A-to-Z listing of whole foods.)

WHOLE FOODS: THE LETTER *A*

abiu	American mayapple
açaí	Anaheim chile
acerola	Ancho chile
ackee	apple
acorn squash	apricot
aduki bean	arame
African cherry orange	araza
agar	arhat
alaria	arrowroot
alfalfa	artichoke
algae	arugula
alligator apple	asafetida
almonds	Asian pear
aloe	asparagus
amaranth	atemoya
Amazon grape	avocado
ambarella	

Eat (and Drink) Your Veggies

It's really that simple. In the LOVE*Lifestyle, veggies—along with fruits, grains, legumes, nuts, seeds, seaweeds, sprouts, and grasses—are our medicine cabinet, and the idea is that if you eat enough of them, you won't actually have to open a medicine cabinet. As you read through the juicing recipes, you'll learn some fantastic facts about individual vegetables and how your juices, smoothies, and vegetable-based dishes can serve you best at any point in your life. You will be amazed at the range of flavors in the vegetable world, and I promise you will find the LOVE* to be abundant and a most enjoyable experience. No deprivation here!

> **Nothing will benefit human health and increase chances of survival for life on earth as much as the evolution to a vegetarian diet."**
>
> —ALBERT EINSTEIN

Live Enzymes = Energy

Enzymes are tiny proteins (amino acids) that assist in chemical reactions, are present in all living cells, and are the primary motivator of all bodily processes, constantly building and rebuilding our bodies. Life without enzymes simply isn't possible. Think of enzymes as the body's workforce, with millions of enzymes constantly at work in every living cell.

Each food in its raw state contains its own enzymes to help break it down, which means the LOVE*Lifestyle provides enzymes aplenty. Enzyme-rich living foods take the burden off an overloaded system and allow it to recover. The food of LOVE* contains its own digestive enzymes, so the body does not have to use its own supply; in fact, they begin to digest the food before the digestive process even begins by breaking down the molecular bonds in food and making the food small enough to pass into the bloodstream.

When it comes to maintaining enzymes, temperature is an all-important factor. Enzymes are very sensitive to heat: They work within limited tempera-tures, 92° to 104°F, close to body temperature, and start to transform or change above 118°F, which is why LOVE* foodies following a high-raw diet don't heat their food above 118°F; anything over that temperature is no longer considered raw, live, or enzymatically active. And it's not just the loss of a few enzymes: When we eat cooked foods, our bodies wind up using their *own* enzymes to do the digestion, meaning the body is working harder and harder with a constantly diminishing supply. And then it's a downward spiral, with enzymes fading faster as we age, resulting in weakened digestion and a quickening of the aging pro-cess. Oh my!

Think of the LOVE*Lifestyle as an enzyme support program, or the lazy per-son's guide to enzyme maintenance. Your body simply has less work to do in the enzyme-making department.

Alkalize to Eliminate Ailments

Alkalinity is the new buzzword, for good reason. Most people intuitively under-stand the concept of alkaline versus acid, and that there's a balance our bodies require for optimal health. A slightly alkaline pH, 7.365 to be exact, is where our blood needs to stay; tiny fluctuations down (the lower the pH, the more acidic we are) can have a large effect on our health.

[11]

Our modern lifestyles are laden with acid contributors, and favoring cooked foods from our industrial food system is acidifying; put another way, a high-cooked diet is a shortcut to acidic ills such as digestive distress, chronic fa-tigue, inflammation, breakdown of body systems, and chronic illness.

We need to replenish our alkaline supply via our diet. Our blood will do everything necessary to keep its alkaline pH, but if the elimination channels are blocked (think constipation, lack of circulation, not sweating, dehydration), those acids are thrown back into the tissues. And if you keep pushing your acidic ways, you will tax your mineral supply (your bones, muscles, and teeth).

Those minerals are called upon when dietary alkalinity is not available to neutralize and balance the acid levels. If these conditions of stress continue, you are looking at inflammation, degeneration, the C-word, or worse. Definitely expect symptoms such as aches and pains at the best, and some of those other scary words at the worst.

If you'd like to go easier on yourself and live by your alkaline design—as Dr. Robert O. Young, author of *The pH Miracle,* would say—favor living alkaline foods. Knowing that, you'll be pleased to learn that most foods on Organic Avenue's LOVE*Lifestyle approach to eating are alkaline forming. Some experts recommend an ideal balance of 80 percent alkaline-forming foods and 20 percent acid-forming foods, which is a convenient number because it's the same ratio we generally recommend for raw to cooked food: 80 percent raw to 20 percent cooked.

Start by adding in foods that are alkaline contributors (low-acid fruits: cucumbers, red peppers, avocados, lemons, limes), along with all the vegetables your heart desires. And here are a few simple general rules of thumb: Living foods are just about always more alkaline forming than cooked foods. Vegetables are moderately to maximally alkalizing in their raw state. Sweeter fruits can be acid forming, but less so if you eat them raw. High-protein foods, particularly meat and dairy, and sugar, tend to be acidifying, which is one reason we avoid them in the LOVE*Lifestyle. And when you're feeling less than excellent, step up your alkaline percentage from 80 to closer to 100 percent for a health boost.

Go Green for Glory with Chlorophyll

Green is great! It's the color of the heart chakra, the color of money, and the color of chlorophyll. Chlorophyll is the pigment found in the leaves of plants, and it is just as vital as the heart and even more valuable than money.

Think of chlorophyll as liquid gold: the energy of the sun in plant form, with benefits such as supporting healthy blood, building a balanced pH body, regenerating and cleansing the body at the cellular level, and improving the health of all the body systems. So if you want to make sure your red blood cells are working their best, turn to the power of the sun. Now, how do you get more chlorophyll? You guessed it: Eat your greens, and drink them too, with green juices such as Cleansing Chlorophyll Booster Shot (page 111) and Wowing Wheatgrass Booster Shot (page 112), be it during one of the LOVE*Cleanses or as you transition back and maintain the radiant health you've found along the LOVE* journey.

A WORD ABOUT WHEATGRASS

Grass, the humble blades below our feet, is often overlooked, its intense nutrient and blood-building chlorophyll content passed by. Wheatgrass juice is a common staple in health food stores, and a healthy daily dose will keep your cells happy.

Here's why: One ounce of wheatgrass juice contains more than one hundred vitamins, minerals, and amino acids and has the nutritional value of more than two pounds of fresh green vegetables. It is also very high in vitamins A, B complex, C, and E. It contains beta-carotene, which acts to ward off the effects of pollution and other toxins. Wheatgrass cleanses, purifies, and boosts the immune system. It has a long tradition as a blood cleanser and powerful detoxifying agent, it helps to increase enzyme levels in the body, builds red blood cells, aids digestion, and stimulates and regenerates the liver. When you're looking for a quick delivery of superfood, you can't do better than a shot of wheatgrass. Make it a double!

[13]

Sprout It

Want to get the biggest nutritional punch from your food? Sprout it! Sprouts are packed with more nutrients per calorie than any other food, and they are tops in protein. Sprouts are also rich in minerals, vitamins, trace elements, antioxidants, and chlorophyll. Eating sprouted foods activates enzymes and predigests complex nutrient structures including protein, fat, and carbohydrates. Sprouts are a superfood (see opposite).

Sprouts take the word *living* to a whole new level. Why? Because when you sprout, you start with an already-healthy live food (cooked food will not sprout) and bring to it even more living qualities. Just soak the nut, seed, grain, or legume overnight, drain, place in a sprouting jar, cover with cheesecloth (to keep air circulating but bugs out), and leave for one to five days; rinse daily until your food grows a little tail. Now that food has even more of what it had to begin with: vitality, minerals, life! For example, when oats are sprouted, the vitamin B_2 level increases by 1300 percent, vitamin B_6 increases by 500 percent, and folic acid by 600 percent. Wow!

Whenever someone asks me about protein, sprouts are what come to mind. Sprouts are an overlooked nutritional powerhouse. If you can develop a sprout habit or add sprouts to your juicing habit, congratulations: You have just excelled on your path to LOVE*. You will receive so much value for the pennies spent on sprouting—and sprouting at home costs, literally, just pennies a day. Rather than feeding farm animals those seeds and grains, we could feed the world with this valuable form of protein, making more efficient use of our resources, especially our precious water, as we do so.

How can you use your sprouts? Blend them into smoothies, juice them, enjoy them on your salads, top your soup with them, include some in a collard wrap or sandwich, or toss them with oil and salt to munch on at the movies as you would popcorn.

Superfoods

We all like to get where we're going, and get there fast. Which explains the current superfood craze. Superfoods are quick, potent nutrition delivery vehicles in the journey of health. But which foods are superfoods? While *superfood* is not a precise scientific term, superfoods are generally considered to be foods that are particularly high in vitamins, minerals, and phytochemicals. Many superfoods are naturally low in calories, so you can eat a lot of them. The LOVE*Lifestyle considers many of our live fruits, vegetables, seaweeds, and sprouts to be superfoods: As we've just learned, living foods are rich in chlorophyll and enzymes and promote an alkaline body, and that, simply put, is super! So follow the LOVE* and you're good to go without getting bogged down about whether this or that vegetable or fruit technically is a superfood and how high it is ranked. They're all good! You might want to keep a lookout for or special order some of these:

[15]

açaí berry	Incan berries
acerola cherry	kelp
barley grass	maca powder
cacao nibs	mangosteen
camu camu	maqui
chaga mushrooms	noni
chia seeds	red pine needle oil
chlorella powder	supergreen powders
coconut oil	wheatgrass powder

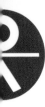

O = Organic

The word is our first name, so you bet we're serious about the importance of organic farming! The USDA organic labeling rules are pretty stringent—no pesticides, synthetic fertilizers, sewage sludge, genetically modified organisms, or ionizing radiation—but keep in mind that the USDA only requires that a product be at least 95 percent organic (and the "made with organic" label requires only 70 percent organic ingredients). At Organic Avenue, we like to go a few steps further. We are constantly in touch with our farmers and producers and maintain relationships with only those who are using the best, most sustainable practices. You can do this too by favoring farmers' markets and getting to know the people who help you put food on your table: Local and organic is something to go for whenever possible.

Why does organic matter so much to us? For starters, the Environmental Protection Agency considers 60 percent of herbicides, 90 percent of fungicides, and 30 percent of insecticides to be carcinogenic, and many are linked to reproductive system dysfunction and nervous system damage. Just reading that makes me nervous! And it's not just about what's added to nonorganic food, but also what's lacking, as nonorganic food comes up short in the nutrition department. A 2008 review of ninety-seven published studies by the Organic Center concluded that organic plant-based foods contain higher levels of several vitamins, including vitamins A, C, and E, and higher concentrations of polyphenols, antioxidants, flavonoids, essential fatty acids, and minerals. The study found organic produce to be 25 percent more nutrient dense than nonorganic produce.

If cost is an issue, favor organic produce from the Environmental Working Group's "dirty dozen," twelve fruits and vegetables that in their nonorganic form consistently are found to have the highest levels of pesticide residue: apples, celery, bell peppers, peaches, strawberries, nectarines (imported), grapes, spinach, lettuce, cucumbers, blueberries, and potatoes (green beans and kale have recently been added to the list in a new "plus" category). When you go for the LOVE*, you'll most likely find yourself preparing meals in your own kitchen more often and consciously choosing what goes into your body rather than randomly grabbing something from the nearest deli; this change in behavior is an immediate cost saver. Organic produce on average is about 20 percent more expensive than nonorganic produce, but if you consider that it's 25 percent more nutritional, in a sense organic works out to be cheaper.

> **❝ Taste the LOVE*, eliminate the hunger. Not only does the Live. Organic. Vegan. Experience. solve the health and the environmental challenges of today, you can help eliminate your body's starvation for the vital nutrients that construct you."**
> —DENISE MARI

[17]

Genetic Modification: Nothing Conventional About It

Once upon a time some of us would tackle nonorganic produce by peeling it to rid it of pesticide residue. But now, thanks to genetic modification, pesticides have been spliced into the seeds of nonorganic, aka "conventional," produce, so there is no avoiding it. Strange how putting chemicals inside the food we eat became something "scientifically advanced," yet in the natural world we are watching as everything from monarch butterflies to our precious pollinating bees comes closer to extinction . . . perhaps with us not too far behind them. OMG—GMOs!

Fortunately, a self-educated bunch have been fighting the good fight to keep

GMOs out of organic foods, so we still have a choice. It's not an easy battle, as the big bucks are ready to spend to move their science experiments forward. Yet Organic Avenue, by adopting the USDA organic certification and continuing to support organic farmers, has kept its purity and its name. After all, it's how we eat and drink, and we think others should at the very least be given a choice to do so as well.

A Numbers Game: How to Identify Organic Produce

The first number on the PLU code of your produce tells you how it was grown:

9: Organic
3 or 4: Nonorganic/conventional
8: Genetically modified

Knowing your numbers isn't quite enough, though: Because labeling genetically modified foods as such is completely voluntary, the absence of an 8 doesn't imply non-GMO. A bit of inverse logic for you there. And food suppliers aren't particularly forthcoming with GMO labeling, as most Americans say they would avoid GMOs if they were labeled (look for changes, though; a groundswell for GMO labeling is growing as I write!). Be particularly careful when it comes to corn and favor the number 9, as genetically modified sweet corn has recently made it into the market unlabeled.

Taste It!

Top chefs and lovers of good food agree that organic produce simply tastes better than nonorganic produce. According to the Organic Center, 43 percent of consumers choose organic because of taste. As organic produce is grown in rich, well-balanced soil, logic would tell us that this would be the case. Try a taste test and see for yourself!

Choosing Organic, a Choice for the Earth

Entire books have been written on the importance of organics, and I encourage you to explore the subject as much as possible. For now I'll leave you with a final big-picture point to ponder: When you choose organic, you are choosing to protect the earth. Organic farming helps prevent soil erosion and mineral and nutrient depletion, saves our water from pollution, and conserves energy. I like to think of it as a life insurance policy for the planet.

[19]

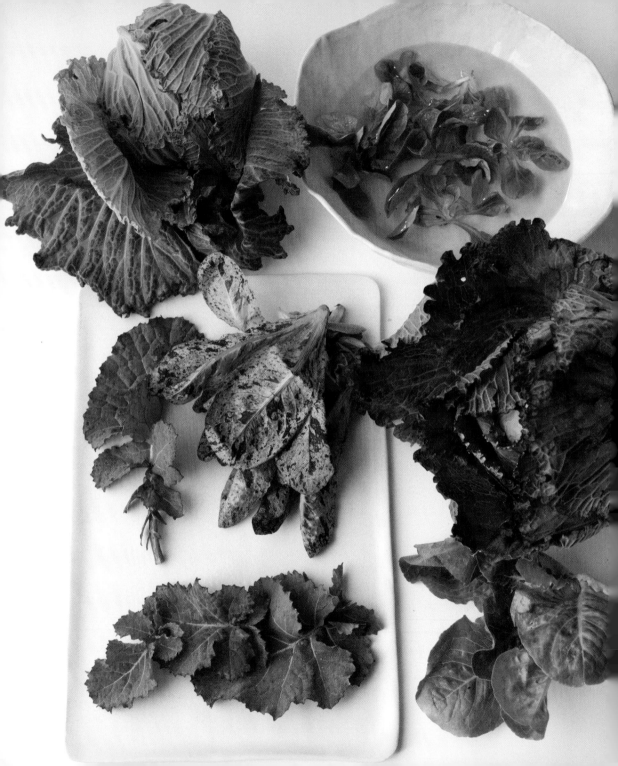

V = Vegan

As I talked about in the beginning of this chapter, LOVE* is not just about being a vegan but rather the desire to live a joyful, happy existence and to allow all beings on the planet to do the same, to follow an ahimsa (nonviolent) lifestyle as much as possible. But there is no LOVE* without veganism, and for purposes of definition, a **vegan** is someone who eats plant-based products (whether grown on land or in the water). The vegan focus is to not live at the expense of the exploitation of animals, so vegans exclude all animal products: meat, fish, dairy, and eggs; vegans generally do not eat honey, either. And vegan consciousness is not just about the food we eat but the materials we buy: Vegans stay away from products that are derived from animals, such as leather, wool, cashmere, and silk, and beauty products such as cosmetics and soaps that are tested on animals. Many people become vegans because they are compassionate toward animals, and some also believe that animal production is an inefficient way of turning out food, one our heavily populated world cannot continue to sustain. Losing weight and maximizing health are other draws for becoming a vegan. Just ask Bill Clinton, Ellen DeGeneres, Alicia Silverstone, Carrie Underwood, Ted Danson, Russell Simmons, Kristin Bell, Christie Brinkley, Olivia Wilde, Stella McCartney, Toby Maguire, Brandon Brazier, Cory Booker, Woody Harrelson, Alec Baldwin, Sandra Oh, Moby . . . the list goes on.

As I've mentioned, vegans learn to get curious about our food sources and to be astute label readers. Earlier I talked about hidden animal products found in what we might assume are vegan foods: bone char to whiten white sugar and dairy in soy cheese. A few more unsuspecting examples: dairy-based lactic acid found in some sauerkraut and pickles, gelatin made from animal or fish bones in nonvegan marshmallows, egg whites sometimes used to clarify wine, and the bizarre beetle-derived red dye in maraschino cherries. Sometimes these ingredients aren't included in the ingredient list, so if in doubt, a call to the manufacturer is the way to go. And remember that labels often change, so check the same label periodically for subtle or not so subtle changes. Look for the letter "V" on the label; anything else may be questionable. A nice side benefit of all that label reading: Once you become more familiar with what goes into your food, you are more likely to choose the best-quality, most nutritious vegan products on the shelves.

TAKE IT FROM THE BEES
Honey is a perfect food—if you are a bee. But if you heat that honey and feed it to those bees, it will kill them. Interesting.

The Protein Question

"Where do you get your protein?" is an inevitable question we vegans often get. Surprisingly, the amount of protein that we need is a lot less than we might think, and key in the protein conversation is the subject of amino acids.

Earlier we learned that enzymes work to build our bodies and that they are made from amino acids. Enzymes do the building, while amino acids, which are the individual components of protein chains, are the materials used for the building: a dynamic duo if ever there was one. This is the order in which protein in the body is formed: (1) Our bodies take in protein, (2) our bodies break down that protein into the component amino acids, and (3) our bodies then rebuild protein—to make *human* protein.

Amino acids are involved in thousands of bodily functions, including digestion, cell renewal, and normal liver function. There are about twenty amino acids involved in making the different proteins the human body needs. Nine of these are essential for adults: *Essential* amino acids are thus called because the body cannot make them itself; it can get them only from food, so they must be part of our diets. A deficiency in just one of these essential amino acids can start to break down muscle and put the body out of whack.

Where to get your aminos? All types of proteins—animal and vegetable—are made up of the same amino acids. So you can get all the aminos that you need from either animal or vegetable sources. A while back there was a lot of concern about vegetarians getting their "complete protein" in every meal: It was thought that various vegetable proteins had to be mixed in the same meal—rice and beans, for example—to give us all we need. While vegans do need to mix their protein sources to get the full profile of aminos, it turns out that our bodies store amino acids in the blood for several hours, so if we don't get all eight of our aminos in one meal, we can make them up at another meal to complete the profile. (Notable exceptions are quinoa, amaranth, buckwheat, hemp, soy, spirulina, and most sprouts: They are complete vegetable proteins.) And even though most meats are complete proteins all on their own, we consider the plant kingdom to be a better source because plant protein is easier to assimilate than the coagulated protein found in cooked meat, which takes more energy to process, not to mention the health risks that come along with eating meat.

❝ *If slaughterhouses had glass walls, everyone would be a vegetarian."*
—**PAUL McCARTNEY**

Amino Acids: Your Essential Nine

Most of us vegans are familiar with the high-protein plant-based foods: grains, beans, soy, nuts, and seeds, but now that we know how important our essential amino acids are, let's get familiar with what they do and discover some examples of where you can get them in the plant world. Then mix and match to complete the picture for your complete protein!

Essential Amino Acid	What You Need It For	Some of the Places You'll Find It
Histidine	to promote growth	alfalfa, apples, beets, carrots, celery, cucumbers, garlic, pomegranates, radishes, spinach
Isoleucine	blood sugar regulation, muscle production and repair after workouts	almonds, coconut, lentils, olives, papaya, sunflower seeds, walnuts
Leucine	muscle protein synthesis, growth hormone production, and immune system support	almonds, coconut, lentils, olives, papaya, sesame seeds, walnuts
Lysine	calcium absorption, bone development	amaranth, beets, carrots, celery, cucumbers, green beans, lentils, spinach, turnip greens
Methionine	fat metabolism, digestion	apples, cabbage, cauliflower, garlic, pineapple, whole grains

[24]

Essential Amino Acid	What You Need It For	Some of the Places You'll Find It
Phenylalanine	to support mood and brain function	almonds, avocados, beets, carrots, lima beans, pineapple, seeds, spinach, tomatoes
Threonine	antibody production	alfalfa, beans, carrots, collards, kale, lettuce, nuts, papaya, seeds
Tryptophan	to regulate sleep, mood, and appetite	alfalfa, carrots, celery, dates, oats, turnip greens
Valine	muscle metabolism, tissue repair, nitrogen balance	apples, beets, carrots, celery, grains, mushrooms, pomegranates, tomatoes

[25]

" *You can be a part of the solution, a solution that is creating a world where farmland is used to feed people, not cattle or other animals being fattened up to fatten you. It's a lovely thing to know you are not directly harming another—or harming yourself!"*

—DENISE MARI

Now that we've covered our aminos, how much protein do we in fact need? Not so much, it turns out: While the USDA requirements are 56 grams a day for men and 46 grams for women, the World Health Organization says that Americans on average actually get about 50 percent more protein than they need. The WHO recommendation is 5 percent of calories from protein for both men and women. (Infants' first food, breast milk, is 5 percent protein.) This means about 38 grams of protein for a man eating 3000 calories a day and 29 grams for a woman eating 2300 calories a day. The 5 percent figure is what much of the world eats, but in Western countries we tend to have a more-is-better approach to protein, with a veritable protein free-for-all for those favoring current high-protein, low-carb diets.

Eating too much protein has its risks, as experts in the field such as Dr. John McDougall and T. Colin Campbell, author of *The China Study,* have shown us through their research. Dr. Campbell tells us that different proportions of amino acids in animal proteins is not always a good thing: Meat has a higher concentration of sulfur-containing amino acids, which metabolize to sulfuric acid, meaning animal protein can throw our pH balance in the acidic direction. Other risks of a meat-based diet include impaired kidney and liver function, calcium excretion that can lead to weakening of the bones and osteoporosis, and heart disease. Protein-heavy diets often don't leave enough room for other food groups like vegetables and are notoriously low in fiber, vitamins, and minerals and high in saturated fat and calories: a SAD (standard American diet) picture.

[26]

❝ We all love animals. Why do we call some 'pets' and others 'dinner'?"

—k.d. lang

Be Free with Fat (Raw Plant Fat, That Is)

Fat is a good thing, if you know how to do fat right. Our brain is mostly fat (about 60 percent), and the myelin sheath, the fatty coating of the brain cells, is mostly fat. So if you value your brain, make sure to lubricate it with some good fats. You also need fats to maintain energy; keep your skin, hair, and nails in top form; keep your stress in check and your mood a positive one; and generally keep all systems in working order. You literally can't live without fat.

Fat cushions you from falls, it keeps you warm, and most of all it guards you against acidic toxins that make their way into your bloodstream and are buried deep away in the fatty tissues when not properly eliminated. Yes, fat is protecting you! Fat is also an excellent slow-burning energy source: When you are on the LOVE* diet, you can eat abundantly of raw, plant-based fats and appreciate beautiful results: healthy skin and connective tissue, flexibility, and just the right amount of softness. You won't have to worry about becoming fat when you eat the right types of fats; just shift your acid ways in the alkaline direction (see page 11) and watch the extra fat on your body melt away. If you feel your body is holding on to fat, step up your level of raw alkaline eating: Your body will keep only the fat it needs to protect it from whatever level of acid your current lifestyle is contributing.

All that said, the type of fat you favor makes all the difference. So how do you do fat right? Get it from cholesterol-free (yep, no animal = no cholesterol) plant-based sources following the LOVE* way of eating. Think avocados, olives, nuts, and seeds. Cold-pressed olive oil, hemp seed oil, flaxseed oil, and avocado oil. Oils retain their quality best when stored in dark glass bottles away from heat and light.

Favoring raw fats—untoasted nuts and unheated oils—as much as possible is the way to go, as fats change their chemical composition when they are cooked, kind of like a mad science project. The canola oil that your chips are fried in? Don't believe the health hype. Those omega-3s oxidize at temperatures

[27]

above 100°F, which starts the process of free radical formation and makes the oil a potential carcinogen. In fact, any omega-3-containing foods degrade under conditions of heat, which gives pause to the current recommendation to include a serving of broiled salmon in your dinner rotation. (Hmm . . . maybe just another misguided recommendation, not unlike "drink cow's milk"—even though you are a human?)

If you are consciously cooking some of your foods, try adding your oil *after* cooking to keep the oil raw. Or use heart-healthy, metabolism-boosting virgin coconut oil, as it's low in omega-3 fatty acids and heat stable, which means it doesn't degrade when heated to relatively high temperatures.

> ❝ *What if eating meat wasn't necessary to produce a healthy, happy human being. Would you still do it?"*
>
> —DENISE MARI

Don't Forget About Fiber

Vegetable fiber is essential. And just as we believe in the power of juice, we also believe in the power of whole food plant-based eating. So the invitation is to load up on fiber-filled veggies; the fiber in those veggies is the bulk that makes elimination easy. Luckily, the food of LOVE* is loaded with fiber. Especially smoothies: A fruit- and vegetable-based smoothie will give you the benefits of eating a large portion of fiber-rich produce in concentrated form. It's a great start to the day . . . and most claim miraculous movements the morning after!

Smart Supplements: For That Extra Bit of Insurance

Thanks to our fast-paced, high-stress modern lifestyle, diet alone often isn't enough to give our bodies all they need. On any diet, vegan or not, taking a quality multivitamin can be a good thing. Avoid gelatin caps (think boiled horse hooves and other strange things) and find a brand you trust after research and consultation with your health-care practitioner. Make sure your multivitamin contains vitamins B_{12} and D_3 (a vegan version), as these days many people, not just vegetarians, are found to be deficient in these two nutrients. Or better yet, consider taking these two crucial supplements on their own in consultation with your health-care practitioner. To top it off, a flaxseed oil supplement (or a daily spoonful of flax oil) for our omega-3-hungry bodies is a smart way to ensure fatty acid intake.

Search out whole food plant-based supplements rather than synthetic supplements. Why? Because the body was designed to digest foods found in nature and can tell the difference between synthetic and real. Synthetics are not absorbed as well as natural supplements and can deplete your body of other nutrients and, in the case of fat-soluble vitamins such as A, D, and E, result in a toxic buildup. Beware: Supplements can be labeled "natural" if they contain as little as 10 percent of the natural form of the vitamin. Look for recognizable plant food sources on the label. If in doubt, you can't go wrong with a call to the manufacturer.

[29]

> **" Part of my reason for being vegetarian is because it practices respect and love for life all through the day, so three times a day you make a decision to eat things that have not been killed."**
> **—NATALIE PORTMAN**

A Matter of Choice

Most people think cow's milk and supplements when the question of calcium comes up, and animal flesh when thinking of iron and protein, but the truth is that all the essential nutrients you need for strong, healthy bodies are found in the LOVE*Lifestyle whole food plant-based way of eating. You can find bone-building and blood-building nutrients in fresh leafy greens, vegetables, sprouts, and even grasses, and you can find strong cleansers and detoxifiers in the form of fresh fruit juices. No harm, no foul. No need to kill any living creature because of a nutritional need.

The reality is that we have access to the plants that make healthy animals and we have a choice to eat lower on the food chain ourselves for greater health. Yes, it's a choice, and I also believe it's a natural law. So just as that lovely conundrum of free will and karma come into play, we have a choice to eat lower on the food chain, and in return we are rewarded.

We are living in a time of choice. I know what my choice is: LOVE*. What will your choice be?

> ### A MILLION STRONG
> According to the Vegetarian Resource Group, there are about 1 million vegans in the United States.

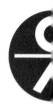

E = Experience

We're at the final letter: The LOVE* is almost complete. The "E" is for tending to not just the food on your plate but the broader picture, too: the physical, mental, and emotional experience. We strive to balance our lifestyle by feeding both the body and the soul. Let's start with the body, and see what can happen when we fill it with "soul" food.

❝ *Faith begins as an experiment and ends as an experience."*

—**W. R. INGE**

Feed Your Body, Feed Your Soul

A level of heightened awareness is one of the things I enjoy most about the LOVE*Foods approach. The physical glow and clear eyes that come with the lifestyle are apparent, but there's a sense of connecting with the energy and the world around you that science may not be able to explain, that you just have to experience. Clarity is felt by many: For me that clarity came as I began to understand my purpose and the role Organic Avenue would play in it, along with many other passions I have that are yet to be converted into projects—not to mention all the books still to be written! What might it mean for you?

I believe that the closer we get to eating from our optimal food source, the more optimal our lives become. While many of the foods on the standard American diet may smell like and look like food, they may leave you functioning on half power (the lights are on but no one's home!). When you experience the LOVE*, the joy of a fully nourished, optimally functioning body, it is, in a word, divine.

Choosing foods with a higher vibration is feeding the soul, and the consciousness you bring to that same food makes a difference. And choosing which foods you're going to spend your money on is an empowering way to have an impact on what you want to see more of on the planet.

If you are feeling depressed or low on energy, now may be a good time to transition to a conscious LOVE*-based diet. (Check out any major symptoms with your health-care provider first.) A diet full of LOVE* is for beginners as well as people who have tried everything. It's for all of us! The change could happen really fast, or it may take a little longer depending on the body, but don't be surprised if an increase in joy, well-being, connectedness, happiness, and energy are the results, with no negative side effects.

Detoxification via Elimination

There are four ways your body physically eliminates its waste and balances itself: respiration, perspiration, urination, and defecation. (And let's not forget vacation for a mental detox program!)

> **Respire:** Breathe. Excite the breath through exercise; relax it through meditation.
> **Perspire:** Run around the block; sweat it out in a sauna or whirlpool or at home in the tub.
> **Urinate:** Stay hydrated.
> **Defecate:** Or, put more delicately, eat plenty of fiber to keep things going.

Elimination keeps your pH balanced and all systems in working order—so take care of all four avenues of elimination to ensure you are shedding unLOVE*ing (aka toxins) on a daily basis.

Often when people cleanse, shift their diet or lifestyle, or even just begin to eliminate "bad" things or add "good" things, cleansing reactions can occur. Over the years of offering the LOVE*Cleanse programs I have received no reports of severe reactions, though it is not uncommon for someone who drinks a daily cup of joe or other caffeinated substance such as tea or soda to have a "cleansing reaction." Caffeine withdrawal is very real and can be managed first by realizing what is likely to happen before it's happening. (I talk more about this on page 44.) If you know your reactions are because you are in a detox state and that it will last only a day or two—or three the most—you are more likely to go with a "this too shall pass" attitude and be rewarded when you allow yourself to experience your own natural energy. And once you feel what it is like to go without, and to eliminate those sleepless nights and anxious days . . . who knows, you just may decide to keep it kicked and roll from there.

Yet beyond the caffeine withdrawal are some other potential side effects to cleansing and rebooting your life depending on how far you have strayed and how long and how well your body was able to eliminate or accumulate toxic substances that were ingested—or became toxic because they weren't eliminated in proper time.

[33]

In many of the old health books on cleansing, you will hear about the infamous "cleansing reactions" and "healing crisis." To make a long story short: Sometimes it gets worse before it gets better. One way to know if you are having a healing crisis is to check with yourself: Were you eating right and exercising and all of a sudden you don't feel well? That just might be a healing crisis, on the brink of a shift into heightened health. On the other hand, if you were drinking, smoking, and eating fried foods and you didn't feel well . . . well, it's just obvious why you aren't feeling well. If you've ever heard someone say they went raw for a week and got sick, it is often that finally the body has been given an opportunity to clean house and it has shifted into cleanse mode, stirring things up as the body expels (to the best of its ability) unLOVE*ing toxins via respiration, perspiration, urination, and defecation. Let your symptoms guide you: Rest when tired, drink when thirsty, and so on. And then there's nothing stopping you from taking on the LOVE*Lifestyle full throttle and remaking your entire being from vibrant, whole, plant-based foods. Just like (I believe) Nature intended.

Exercise

Create some time each day for movement: Do what you love. It's important to build a space for exercise to set the tone that this is something you do to value yourself and your health. A couple of ways are to find an exercise buddy or make a commitment to a certain class. Walking is a great form of exercise, and if you get that going, all of a sudden you may find yourself jogging. Breaking a sweat is a good exercise goal, as sweating is a wonderful way to detox.

I love trying new things, changing them up to make exercise interesting rather than simply a routine. Biking in the city with my son, playing basketball, rebounding (bouncing on a mini trampoline—my favorite), practicing yoga, hiking. You don't have to limit your exercise to the gym, not even here in New York City, where we have miles of car-free space available to explore. Just remember to keep it fun so you can keep it up!

[34]

Meditate

There are many types of meditation worthy of exploration. Vipassana meditation in particular resonates with me; I find it one of the most helpful tools for building a balanced life. This simple Buddhist style of meditation goes back 2,500 years and continues to be a practical tool today. *Vipassana* means "to see things as they really are," and that's what it's all about: self-transformation through self-observation, and ultimately happiness and liberation. There are Vipassana centers throughout the country; you can find them through www.dhamma.org.

A COMMITMENT TO MOVEMENT

It takes thirty days to form a habit. So commit to exercise rain or shine, thirty minutes a day for thirty days, no matter what. Decide that this new dedication to movement is not an option; it is a devotion you will continue from now on. When movement is no longer just for when the weather is perfect, you are free to do anything your heart desires: dance around the house, climb the stairs in your building, or go out and weather the storms and be reborn. Remember when you were a child and you would have given anything to go play in the puddles? Now you can!

Setting your breath in the morning with meditation helps keep the brain oxygenated throughout the day. Start slowly: Try setting the timer on your phone (don't forget to put the ringer on vibrate!) for as little as 3 minutes, work your way to 7 minutes, next 11 minutes, and then sit more if you wish. No pressure. Nothing to do, nowhere to go for those precious minutes.

Sit and watch your breath. Feel it on your nose. Don't try to control it. Recognize your thoughts, release them, and go back to the emptiness.

Next step: Begin to relax your muscles. Start at your head and face, and really notice where you are holding: is it your jaw, your brow? Breathe away the tension, and if you have a thought and realize that the tension is accumulating again, just release again. Continue relaxing your muscles from your head to your toes, all the while being mindful of your breath and releasing thoughts like clouds floating through the blue skies. They come, they go . . . don't hold on to them or give them any more life than they already have. Just let them go, let your physical tension go, and breathe. If you find yourself a little too worked up, try counting silently to yourself to keep the thoughts in check. You will notice the benefits of this simple practice relatively quickly, just as with a LOVE*Cleanse: Generally, three days will bring on the results from your new practice. What might you expect from meditation? An increase in creativity, a sense of calm and clarity, increased self-awareness, more restful sleep, and a feeling of fulfillment are benefits many meditators report from the field. Be open to the unexpected!

> **❝ Meditation is a tool that will bring more LOVE* to the planet."**
> —DENISE MARI

IT'S ALL CONNECTED

You may notice that by eating more alkalizing, less agitating foods in the LOVE*Lifestyle, you find it easier to get into a meditative state. So if you eat well, you can meditate more easily, and when meditating is easier, eating well comes easier, which works out quite nicely. And did you know that the physical practice of yoga is ultimately a preparation for meditation? It's all connected.

Creating and Connecting with Community for Support and Sharing

Rather than becoming isolated in this new and different way of living that is LOVE*, let's strive to create a community of like minds, whether it's across the sea via the Internet or the local sea of people in your neighborhood. Aspire to find work that nurtures your soul, but if your work environment isn't conducive to the lifestyle, seek out community elsewhere: yoga classes, retreats, spiritual groups, volunteer groups, community vegan potlucks, whatever calls to you. Be the LOVE* and realize the love that's all around you.

I'd like to end this section, the start of the LOVE* journey, by reminding you that there are any number of healthy eating and lifestyle practices at your disposal at any point along the way. By breaking down the acronym, you now understand what goes into the Live. Organic. Vegan. Experience. and how these four words form a seamless whole. You know that there's always something to try when you feel your diet or lifestyle needs a little refining; LOVE* takes time and patience, yet small efforts over time can amount to a whole new body, a whole new you! We are talking about a revolution in the way we eat, and this revolution can lead to evolution in both our health and our connection to the world around us. There is no one set path. There are times for big-picture changes and times for taking it slowly. Trust that you know what's best for you.

Now it's time to introduce you to the LOVE*Cleanses. By choosing to cleanse—whether with a one-day starter or an all-green advanced cleanse—you will be upgrading your energy while subtracting toxins from your system and pounds from your waistline. The result: a radiant new you. Let's get started!

[37]

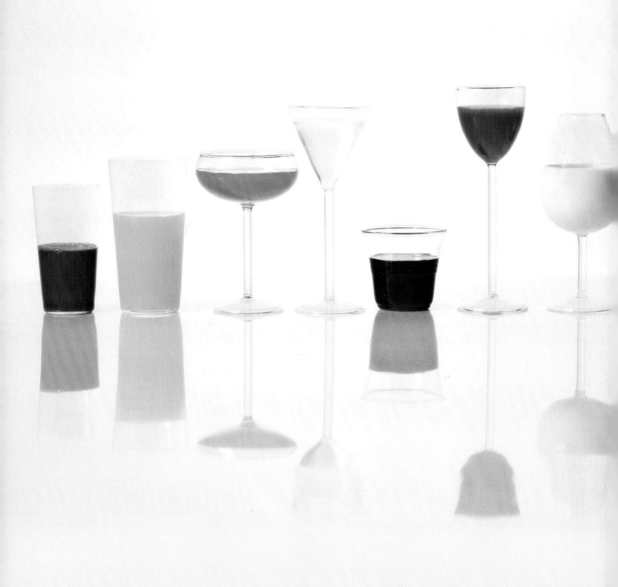

PART II

The LOVE*Cleanse: Cleansing the Organic Avenue Way

Cleansing is a big part of the LOVE*Lifestyle, the very foundation of Organic Avenue, and a great way to kick-start your introduction to this new way of living and eating. Our cells are put under stress daily from a high-sugar acidic diet, negative thoughts and emotions, and a polluted environment. We need a line of defense to combat that stress, which is why many people begin their journey with a juice cleanse and continue with periodic cleanses. This section introduces you to the LOVE*Cleanse, the very same cleanses that we offer at our boutiques. Now you can cleanse the Organic Avenue way from the comfort of your own kitchen—what an empowering and affordable way to take your health into your hands!

First things first, I will explain to you **what LOVE*Cleansing is,** and what makes it such an important tool for finding balance within the body. Then I will go over **the *why* of LOVE*Cleansing,** the powerful case for combating the "unLOVE*ing"—my gentle term for toxins—with liquid nutrition, and what to expect as you undertake this challenge. We need to start somewhere, and for us the key is **starting out smart**—that is, being prepared with the knowledge you need to undertake a successful cleanse. I will give you guidance on what to eat and what to do on the days leading up to your cleanse and the crucial night before. And I'll give the lowdown on **essential equipment** and **ingredients to fill the fridge and pantry.**

When you're ready to start your LOVE*Cleanse, I will **help you choose which one** is best for your needs, from testing the waters with LOVE*Easy to losing weight quickly with LOVE*Deep. I will tell you **what you might expect to feel** while releasing the unLOVE*ing along the way, and **how to deepen your cleanse** with tools such as dry skin brushing and colonics. Helpful tips and inspirational quotes are scattered throughout to keep you motivated every step of the way. Finally, I will give you tips on **how to transition back** into "normal" eating after your cleanse (and you may even find your notion of "normal" eating turned on its head!) and how to maintain the many benefits you've gained along the way. I have also provided a **LOVE*Cleanse FAQ** section, taken from questions we often get from our customers at our boutiques, to set you straight on anything that might need clarification. For some of us, weight loss is a primary goal and we are happy to notice progress in that direction after the very first day of a cleanse. If that's the case for you, you'll be thrilled with secondary effects such as bountiful energy, glowing skin, and more as you continue with your cleanse. This will give you strong incentive to stay the course!

Even if you undertake the challenge of a LOVE*Cleanse for only a short time, I am certain you will be amazed at the sense of clarity and renewed inspiration you'll experience, and more so if you stretch your cleanse further than the typical three to five days. It's a blessing to enjoy and a choice we have today. And once you experience it for yourself, you will likely come back for more. As one of my teachers used to say, "Nothing tastes as good as good health feels." And with the recipes for our popular LOVE*Cleanses now in your hands, it just got that much easier to go for the glory—the Green Glory, that is!

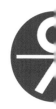

What Is Cleansing?

Remember back in grade-school science class when you learned about homeostasis? We were taught that everything in nature has a tendency to stay pretty much the same under different external conditions, that there's a pull toward equilibrium. Well, that's the game in health, too! Our bodies are designed to naturally rid themselves every day of acidic toxins, what here at Organic Avenue I refer to as the unLOVE*ing elements—chemicals, pesticides, genetically modified organisms, stress hormones, processed food, and artificial additives—as one way to achieve balance. The inner workings of the miraculous body chemistry and our own little internal detoxifying systems (aka organs of elimination: kidneys, liver, lungs, skin, intestines) work to move the accumulated pollution out of the system to keep homeostasis. Activity and rest both have their place in helping the body find its way toward homeostasis, though periods of inactivity, illness, or even dark, cold winters can lead to accelerated breakdown if additional efforts are not put in place as a counterbalance. It's not an onward-upward build-build-build; otherwise our bodies would never stop growing! Balance is the key to sustainable and consistent improvement: It's a slow-and-steady-wins-the-race rather than a radical approach.

To counter the unLOVE*ing forces with a goal toward homeostasis, those on the LOVE*Lifestyle favor organic foods, limit processed foods, drink purified water, and eliminate, reduce, or at the very least manage our intake of caffeine, alcohol, cigarettes, sugar, and other highly acidic substances. Then we introduce nutrient-dense, incredibly alkalizing juices and/or foods that require little work from the digestive system to awaken and begin the heavy hauling: in a word, *cleansing.* The more alkaline contributors you enlist via rest, de-stress, and dedication to a mineral-rich LOVE*Lifestyle, the more opportunity there is to rid excess acidity and achieve the ever elusive homeostasis. Indeed it's a balancing act.

The body's energy can then focus on removing whatever doesn't belong and work toward health and healing. A renewed, energized, radiant you is what is achieved; results are noticed within the first days and continue to amaze the longer you remain on the journey.

Denise Mari's Top Ten Benefits of Cleansing

1. **Cleansing gives you serious nutrition.** When we speak of cleansing, we mean an abundance of natural, fresh, raw plant-based foods and fresh-pressed juices. Fresh juices deliver a dense dose of nutrients in an easy-to-assimilate form, filling you with renewed energy.
2. **Cleansing hydrates you.** You will easily meet and exceed your hydration goals when you follow the LOVE*Cleanse guidelines, remedying everything from dry, dull skin to aches and pains. Remember, on a LOVE*Cleanse you are also drinking plenty of pure water between your nutritional beverages—preferably alkaline water—the body's best cleansing solvent ever!
3. **Cleansing rests your digestion.** Giving those digestive organs a break means increased efficiency and optimal functioning. Just think . . . if you didn't have to go to work every day, you could catch up on your chores. This is what the body does when it's not overburdened by digestion.
4. **Cleansing takes the weight off.** Optimal and efficient means slim and slender. Yes, occasional hunger may be felt during a cleansing period, but it is not from lack of nutrition. You continue to flood your body with the most optimum fuel, and it quickly does the work to dump out what's not needed, resulting in the more optimal you!
5. **Cleansing elevates your mood.** The energy in raw foods and juices can eliminate fog and depression; sheer bliss is an added bonus reported

by many. Isn't it highly motivating to know that pure plant juices and foods can have such profound results? I think we would all agree it's worth a try before heading for a prescription with many scary potential side effects. Try a LOVE*Cleanse and see if you have a new and brighter outlook on life.

6. **Cleansing gives you structure.** It holds your hand with a plan until you are ready to continue with the lifestyle on your own. My friend Dr. Shawn Miller often says, "With love anything is possible," and when LOVE*Cleansing, this is very true.

7. **Cleansing means renewal.** It enables you to break habits and create new, healthier ones. Even daily addictions can be relieved by a periodic abstinence, giving you clarity and strength.

8. **Cleansing gives you freedom.** No time spent on meal planning means more time to think about the life you want to live—and to go ahead and live it! Sometimes freedom comes when guidelines are set, from knowing you can achieve your goals by staying within simple parameters. Freedom can be found in the act of making decisions. Everything from foods to friends becomes easier to choose.

9. **Cleansing clears your conscience.** Eating and drinking low on the food chain is a personal contribution to peace on the planet. It feels good to do good, and it's easy to do good when it tastes good. Win, win, win!

10. **Cleansing becomes a new tool in your tool belt.** It's something you can turn to again and again when the need arises, all the while incorporating more juices and living foods into your everyday plant-based LOVE* diet.

> **❝ I will form good habits and become their slave."**
>
> —OG MANDINO

Why Cleanse?

Even if you have a squeaky clean, highly alkaline diet, you cannot avoid the unLOVE*ing. These unLOVE*ing elements exist everywhere, not just in our food but in our environment as well. Excess stress is part of the unLOVE*ing too,

[43]

as it can lead to an acidic body when excess "fight or flight" hormones get released. Those unLOVE*ing invaders tend to concentrate in the brain, liver, and gastrointestinal tract and can drain our energy and make us more vulnerable to disease and infection. Since everyone is exposed to the unLOVE*ing, everyone can benefit from detoxification on a periodic basis. Cleansing is the rescue squad: It strengthens us and builds our immunity so we can bounce back in the face of this ongoing barrage.

Now, not every person who cleanses has the goal of wanting clean, waste-free cells. You may simply be curious, want to lose weight, be interested in shifting to a more vegetarian or vegan diet, or be recovering from a serious illness or health condition. Maybe you've seen the celebrities toting their orange Organic Avenue bags and you want to know what it is they are doing that gives them their glow. The reasons to cleanse are many and varied, but the results are often similar: an increase in mental clarity, more energy, weight loss, balanced pH, radiant glowing skin, better digestion, and overall increased well-being. Chronic pains begin to subside. (If you have a serious illness or take any prescribed medications, be ready to discuss your newfound LOVE* with your doctor before proceeding.) You will be amazed at the transformation that occurs in just a few days on a LOVE*Cleanse. Immediately benefits begin to be realized, from a confidence boost as you accomplish each LOVE*Cleanse milestone to the pleasurable reward of feeling and looking your best. Just **do it for the LOVE* of it** and revel in the compliments you will begin to receive.

Organic Avenue's Top Ten Transition-to-Cleansing Tips

1. **Gradually wean yourself from caffeine.** Repeat: "This too shall pass." Give yourself three days; your headaches will gradually disappear and you will begin to know true, sustainable energy. Try to transition gently, experimenting with lower-in-caffeine teas instead of coffee, or if large is your style, commit to a small. Take one step at a time. It's best to

replace ritualistic habits with new, healthier ones. If you are hitting the local coffee spot, take a detour to the natural foods store (or your local Organic Avenue!) or decide to create a new LOVE*ing ritual of juicing at home. This, too, is very rewarding.

2. **Clear your system of alcohol and up your intake of pure water.** Hey, it's just for today. Don't think about forever on this one: Take it one day at a time. You can do just about anything for twenty-four hours. As with coffee, the alcohol habit can be overcome in steps too. If a vodka on the rocks is your style, choose to move toward Mighty LOVE* Green Juice (page 127) on the rocks to get some good veggie nutrition into that drink. Increase the juice, decrease the booze. Your skin will thank you for it, as alcohol is very dehydrating (think wrinkles and you may think twice about that drink).

3. **Start incorporating a daily morning fruit juice and an afternoon green juice.** What could be easier than this? Step-by-step, add in the good. Adding in will automatically push out something else less favorable, as there is only so much one can consume each day. Every new addition of a juice means one less coffee, beer, or other devoid-of-nutrition choice.

4. **Peacefully part ways with cigarettes.** If you've picked up a bad habit to deal with frustrating situations, think of replacing it with a good one. My yoga teacher Dharma Mittra calls it fierce determination. If you feel a "fit" come on and want to run to your old go-to hurtful habit, consider doing something positive instead. A friend of mine put down his smokes and opted to replace that cig-response with push-ups. Choose something you can do wherever you are, be it a breathing technique, jumping in place, or stretching. Use positive thoughts to conquer disastrous addictions. You can do it!

5. **Pass on the red meat if you're not already a vegetarian.** It's a good place to start. Though all meats (and even fish) deliver cholesterol and animal hormones, most also contribute chemicals from the unLOVE*ing foods and medicines the animals are fed. It's a bloody mess! Call it what it is. You will be surprised (as I have been) how easy it is to give up red meat. Watch the movie *Earthlings* beginning to end. That should be the end of

that! And, yes, protein is important; we just get it from the same places the other vegetarian animals get it from (remember that vegetarians are some of the largest and strongest animals on the planet). There is no shortage of protein in the LOVE*Lifestyle.

6. **Favor vegetarian and vegan meals as much as you can.** Believe me, there are unlimited guilt-free and delicious food choices with no deprivation when you choose this lifestyle. I must have more than a hundred vegetarian cookbooks—the options are unlimited. Look online; learn how to convert a favorite meat-based recipe to a vegan one. You will be pleasantly surprised at the satisfaction received from an old favorite turned LOVE*ing.

7. **Learn some basic healthy-cooking techniques such as steaming vegetables and some easy dressing recipes.** The way I began to eat veggies was by making sure I had something to dress them with or dip them in. Steaming helps us ease into raw veggies, and a simple finish of olive oil, sea salt, and lemon goes a long way toward making our veggies that much more enjoyable. (I'm getting hungry just writing this!) Use one of our dips (pages 225 to 229) or any of the salad dressing recipes (pages 195 to 211). You can smother those veggies as you're developing a new love for them—that's what I did.

8. **Replace refined carbohydrates like wheat pasta with whole grains.** Or check out the varieties of alternative pastas: rice pasta, quinoa pasta, mung bean pasta, sweet potato pasta, black bean pasta, and so on. Leave processed wheat products behind and continue to enjoy noodles galore.

9. **Dedicate yourself to an exercise program.** For me, first thing in the morning is best. This way no matter what happens with my day I get the exercise in. And if the day allows follow-up with an evening routine, all the better. A great walk is all you need, but as you get more and more fit, you will want to do more. Find hills and pick up the pace. Get your heart beating! Become increasingly aware of your body, take notice of where you need more toning, and choose exercises that shape you.

10. **Begin utilizing enemas or colonics as part of a healthy lifestyle practice.**
Yes, this might seem strange for some, which is part of the problem with
our modern lifestyle: We've set aside some of the health and hygienic
tools of the past, and now is when we need them more than ever. See
pages 88 to 89 for more on the subject.

See pages 88 to 89 for more on the subject.

A WORD ON WATER

At Organic Avenue, we filter our water to make it alkaline in pH to
counter our acid-forming highly active and stressful lifestyles. At
our stores we sell bottles of high alkaline water and natural spring
water, and at home you'll find my fridge stocked with it. At-home
units like the Watermark, Kangen, or Chanson are recommended.

If you're not buying dedicated alkaline water, I recommend
using a filtration system such as the H2O Nano-Filtration System
for your tap water if you intend to drink it. Go a step further
than the pitcher filters if you can; they perform some stages of
filtration, but multistage filtration systems that attach to the pipes
or faucet have multiple levels. While removing some contaminants
is far better than removing none, why not go for the healthiest
water possible? A good unit will cost you more up front, but if
you refill your eco-friendly bottles, think of all the money you'll
be saving, how much less waste you'll be putting into the system,
and all the good you'll be doing for your body.

[47]

Starting Out Smart: Preparing for Your Cleanse

How should you get ready for your cleanse? It all depends on your personality
type: Some jump right in, some like to prepare. Both work. Most important is
to start out smart, and the best thing you can do to get ready is to incorporate
more fresh and organic raw food, juices, smoothies, soups, and nut mylks into

your everyday diet. This is a wonderful habit that we can all develop. If you don't currently eat a plant-based diet, for optimal results, remove meat, dairy, and all processed foods from your diet on the days leading up to your cleanse. Incorporate fresh, organic vegetable juices and smoothies for breakfast, energizing raw soups and salads for lunch, and a hearty raw salad with gently steamed veggies for dinner. You could also include cooked winter squash, sweet potatoes, or alkaline grains such as quinoa and millet in your dinner meal if cooked food is part of your diet.

The days before your cleanse is when the preparation gets more specific.

Three Days Before You Begin Your LOVE*Cleanse

- Abstain from drinking coffee, or at least cut down considerably. Shift from black or green caffeinated teas to herbal teas. Best to do this ahead of the LOVE*Cleanse itself for an easier experience. Letting go completely during the cleanse may make things a little more challenging during the first one to three days. The hydration from the juices and added water will help during the detox. Caffeine habituation/addiction is very real. Headaches and moodiness are the most common complaints. Take it easy. Know that this too shall pass.
- Avoid all refined (white and brown) sugar, refined salt, and processed foods. (Oops! Did I just remove all your daily foods? Yikes! If so, head to the natural food store and discover the salad bar for an interesting smorgasbord of new foods to try. Go for vegan whole food items and make this a fun learning experience of experimenting with new foods.)
- If you are not a vegetarian or vegan, eliminate or limit greatly your intake of meat, fish, eggs, and dairy. Ideally add in legumes, greens, and veggies, but also feel free to explore vegan "meats" for texture, tofu to replace eggs, and the various mylks from soy, almond, and rice as well as today's wildly improved vegan cheeses (Daiya and Teese brands are my favorites).
- Continue your normal workout regimen. (Or begin one.)

- Consider adding a relaxing bath in the evenings and an herbal tea for a nightcap.
- Continue drinking plenty of filtered water.
- Consume a cleansing menu consisting of fresh, organic fruits and vegetables. Include green juices, wheatgrass juice, green smoothies, and blended vegetable soups if you can; this will greatly facilitate the cleansing process and set the stage for the days ahead.

The Night Before You Begin Your LOVE*Cleanse

- Eat a large green leafy salad with a wide variety of raw vegetables (no beans or grains) or lightly steamed vegetables. Fresh lemon or lime juice, high-quality cold-pressed olive or avocado oil, and sea salt can be added in small amounts. The fiber in the salad will sweep the intestines and prepare the body for fasting.
- Write down your intentions, what you would like to release from your life. When we fast or cleanse, we not only detoxify our organs but also cleanse emotions from the system, giving us the potential to shift unwanted ideas, people, circumstances, and patterns and move into a lighter, more vibrant way of being. Go ahead and list your own intentions here:

[49]

_____

_____

_____

_____

_____

_____

Here are some that have worked for me:

- I am releasing the unLOVE*ing accumulation of toxins in my body.
- I am releasing negativity from my relationships.
- I am releasing my reactive behavior and initiating proactive behavior.
- I am releasing "can't do" and replacing it with "can do"!

Commit to quit: Never give up on giving up! Write a list of all the things you want to change or give up, then add a date or timeline and ideas on how you can start realizing these goals. Then put the paper away. You will be surprised that if you just write down your goals, the Universe just may make them real for you."

—DENISE MARI

JUICE TO JUMP-START

If you want to feel better fast, juice! It's easy, it's delicious, and it will give you the quickest nutritional boost while increasing your energy as the unLOVE*ing elements, aka toxins, are removed and your digestive system and all other systems in the body are renewed.

Live juices are a direct transmission of pure liquid nutrition, as they are loaded with easily absorbable vitamins, minerals, enzymes, purified water, protein, carbohydrates, and the magical chlorophyll. This fiberless form of food (don't worry, you'll be getting plenty of fiber when you eat your veggies) gives many of the benefits of eating without the bulk, making juices a key component of the LOVE*Lifestyle.

Juicing, whether on a LOVE*Cleanse or as an everyday elixir, can be a satisfying experience, even meditative. Make it fun. Enjoy the colors, the smells, and the taste of the different vegetable and fruit juices. Pure pleasure.

Some think that there's too much cleanup involved in home juicing, but if you get into a groove and make it a daily habit, you can find ways to speed up the process (for example, by preparing vegetables beforehand and cleaning as you go). See Readying Your Kitchen for Cleansing on the following pages for advice on choosing a juicer and pages 115 to 151 for the complete Organic Avenue juice recipes.

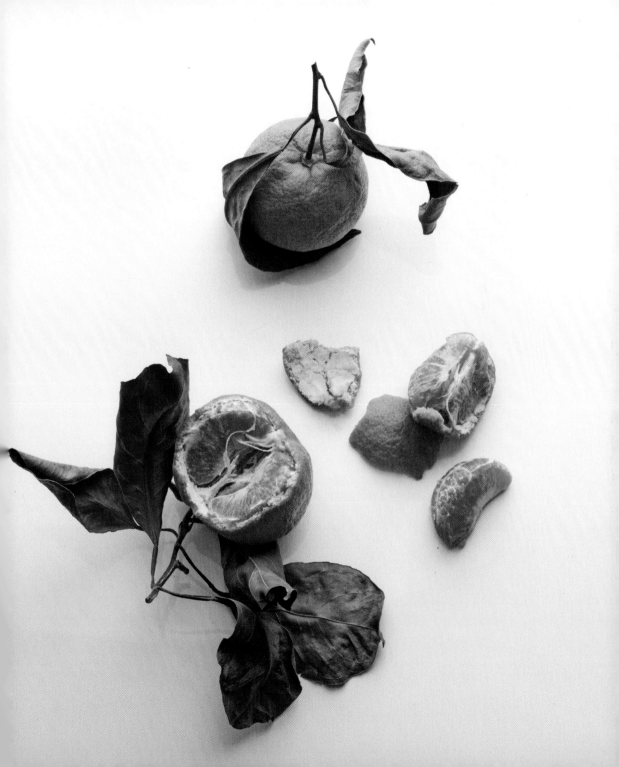

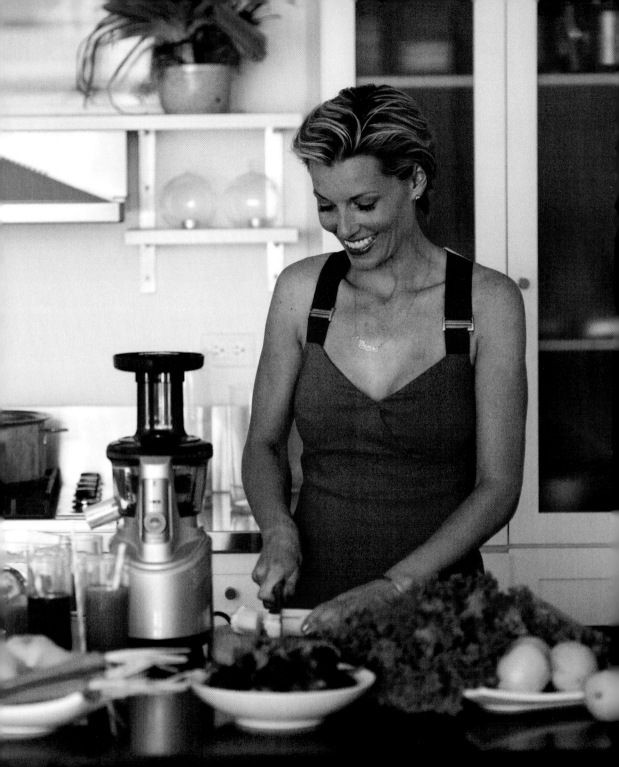

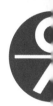

Readying Your Kitchen for Cleansing: Essential Equipment

A few strategic purchases are all you need to set the stage for cleansing and preparing the recipes that you'll find later in this book. I'll give you some guidance here, and I encourage you to do your own research, shop around, and fill your kitchen with the brands you love. And when you find something that does the job, stick with it.

[53]

First and foremost, you'll need a juicer for juicing and a blender for smoothies and nut mylks. How to choose? It depends on your needs, whether you're an occasional cleanser or a LOVE* devotee, and the budget you're working with.

Juicer: Your Number One LOVE*Cleanse Tool

There is a world of juicers out there, widely ranging in price and purpose. I'll describe them for you, then leave you to choose the one that speaks to you. Note that the juices made from these juicers, with the exception of the grind and press, are best enjoyed the day they are made.

Centrifugal Juicer

This the most common everyday juicer, the kind you might find in a department store and with the lowest price point, around $100; Jack LaLanne and Breville are two examples. They work by first shredding your fruits and vegetables, then spinning the pulp, and through centrifugal force they press the pulp against a strainer screen to extract the juice. Greens can be juiced in small amounts, but the centrifugal juicer is best for juicing fruits, making this model a choice for dabblers, the occasional cleanser, and regular fruit juice drinkers.

Masticating Juicer

This juicer grinds (masticates, or chews) and presses the juice in one step, with the juice pouring out the bottom and the pulp ejected separately. In the $250 price range, masticating juicers are more expensive than centrifugal juicers but tend to be sturdier and easily juice both fruits and green vegetables; the pulp comes out drier, and therefore more nutrients are extracted from your produce. Champion and Omega are popular masticating juicers.

Twin-Gear Press

This works in a similar fashion as the masticating juicer, grinding and pressing the juice, but, as it is equipped with two gears that work at slower speeds, it preserves more nutrients than a single-gear auger. It is perfect for large quantities of fibrous greens. At $500 or so, this is an investment, though well worth it for those dedicated to the LOVE*Lifestyle. Green Star is a popular brand.

Grind and Press

This is the king of all juicers, and at more than $2,500, it's for serious juice LOVE*rs. Norwalk is the most common brand, and it's my go-to juicer because of the volume of juice I make. The mineral content of juices from a grind and press is off the charts, significantly more than other juicers. The pulp comes out extremely dry because the maximum amount of juice is extracted; your juice yield will be significantly more with a grind and press (take note of this as you are making the recipes in this book), and those who juice daily can see savings of hundreds of dollars a year in produce bills. And a big plus is that the juice will keep sealed in an airtight container for up to three days without loss of nutrients or flavors.

Blender: Because We LOVE* Our Smoothies

If your blending needs go no further than making nut mylks and the occasional fruit smoothie, a basic model, something your kitchen may already be equipped with, is all you need. A regular blender can take you only so far, though; for those regularly making green smoothies and cheese and yogurt recipes, for example, a high-speed blender is a must. This is why: A high-speed blender takes your recipes to another level of blending. It makes them silky-smooth (emphasis on *silky,* with a little shine to them), beyond what most regular blenders can do. A high-speed blender can even warm up your food, which can come in handy when you're making soups.

[55]

The Vitamix is the go-to high-speed blender for those on the LOVE*Lifestyle, and in the $500 price range, it is a serious investment, but its motor is built to last and will keep the smoothies and soups coming well into the future. A high-speed blender will give you the best results for the recipes in this book.

Food Processor: A Super Sidekick

Much of what you make in a food processor could be made in a high-speed blender, but a food processor can come in handy for shredding and grating vegetables and for blending anything that is more solid than liquid. It's great for making nut butters. A mini food processor is a nice option for occasional use.

Dehydrator: LOVE*-Style Low-Temp "Cooking"

As I mentioned earlier, in order to keep foods live, or raw, we don't heat them above 118°F. But that doesn't mean we can't make cheeses, cookies, and snack foods, just like everyone else! We use a dehydrator to gently transform "raw" ingredients into LOVE*Recipes. The Excalibur is our dehydrator of choice, as it has a thermostat and comes equipped with shelves so you can make several batches of cookies or different recipes of varying sizes and shapes at once. With it are included ParaFlexx sheets, the raw world's version of baking parchment, to line your dehydrator trays. The Excalibur is in the $200 range, more or less, depending on whether you choose a five-tray or a nine-tray model. Having a food dehydrator gives you a wider range of recipes to choose from and keeps things interesting in the kitchen. And if you live in a hot, dry climate, you can try drying your food in the sun (cover it with a mosquito net).

LOVE* Your Accessories

These are some other tools of the trade to complete the LOVE*Kitchen:

- **Chef's knife:** Do some research and buy a brand you love; ceramic knives are my favorite.
- **Nut mylk bags:** For straining your nut mylks; cheesecloth also works well.
- **Sprouting jars:** Use dedicated sprouting jars with mesh screens or simple mason jars (try covering them with cheesecloth or panty hose).

- **Mixing bowls, liquid and dry measuring cups, measuring spoons:** For the best accuracy in following your recipes (though don't be a slave to measurements; once you feel comfortable in the kitchen, experiment and get creative!).
- **Strainers, fine-mesh sieve, cutting board, manual citrus juicer, peeler:** And whatever miscellaneous tools you find you need to complete the picture.

[57]

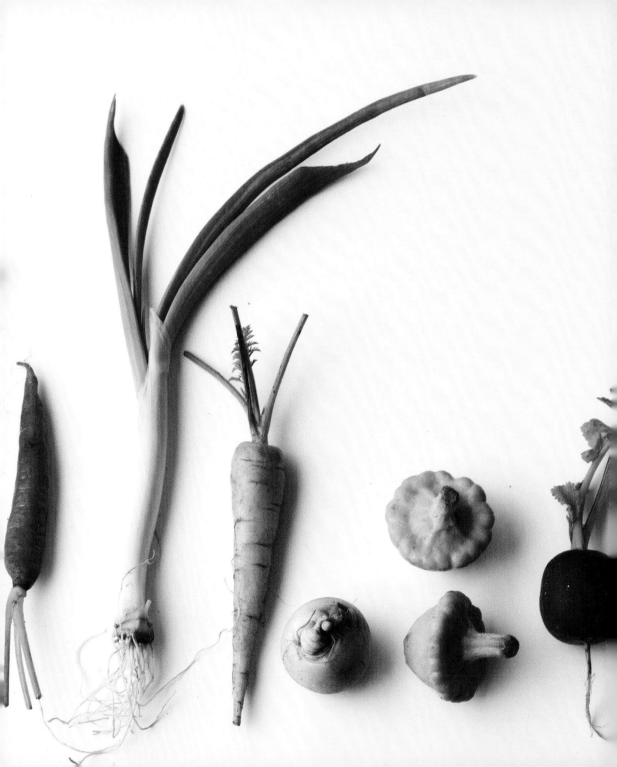

The Ingredients of LOVE*:
Stocking Your Fridge
and Pantry

The LOVE*Kitchen is bountiful, bursting at the seams with green, and 100 percent cruelty-free. These are some of the ingredients that you'll be using as you juice and eat your way into the LOVE*.

The Produce Department: Filling Your Fridge with LOVE*

Vegetables: Arugula, beets, bell peppers, cabbage, carrots, celery, collards, corn, cucumbers, dandelion greens, garlic, jalapeños, kale, lettuce, mushrooms, onions, parsnips, scallions, spinach, Swiss chard, tomatoes, zucchini . . . and whatever you may have harvested from your backyard plot.

Fresh herbs: Basil, cilantro, mint, oregano, parsley. No backyard plot? Try growing herbs in pots on your windowsill.

Fruits: Apples, avocados, bananas, blueberries, grapefruits, lemons, limes, mangos, oranges, pears, pineapple, strawberries . . . and whatever other treasures you find at your local farmers' market.

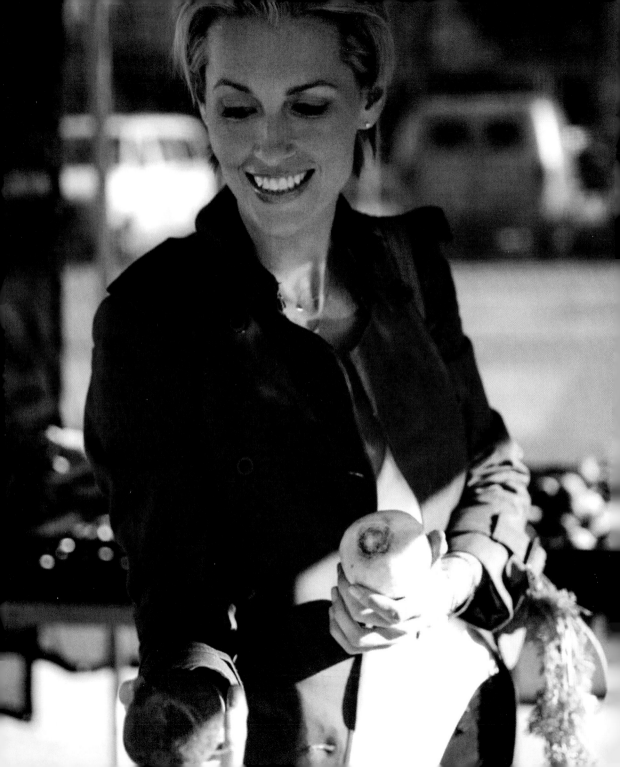

Coconut: A LOVE* of the Fruit in Its Varied Forms

Coconut water: The liquid that comes from a young coconut; found in natural food stores. Unpasteurized coconut water from your natural food store's refrigerated beverage section is a nice convenience.

Coconut meat: The flesh of a young coconut (see page 146 for how to crack 'em).

Shredded coconut: The dried form, for use in dehydrator baking or for sprinkling.

Coconut sugar: A LOVE* low-glycemic sweetener of choice, made from the dehydrated sap of the coconut palm; available from natural food stores or online.

Coconut blossom sugar: A syrup form of coconut sugar; it's lighter in hue than coconut sugar, so it won't affect the color of a recipe.

The Sweet Department

Coconut sugar and coconut blossom sugar (see above).

Lucuma powder: From the lucuma fruit, common to Peru and Chile, known for its caramel flavor and low-glycemic sweetening properties.

Stevia: A noncaloric plant-based sweetener that's up to three hundred times sweeter than sugar, available in liquid or powdered form; use sparingly.

Dried dates: The sweetest fruit there is; they make their way into many a LOVE*Recipe.

[61]

Nuts and Seeds: Foundational Ingredients

Nuts: Almonds, Brazil nuts, cashews, macadamias, pine nuts, pistachios, walnuts.

Seeds: Chia seeds, hemp seeds, pumpkin seeds, sesame seeds, sunflower seeds.

Nut and seed butters: Almond butter, cashew butter, tahini (sesame paste).

Oils, Salt, Dried Herbs and Spices, and Sundry Flavorings

Oils: Extra-virgin olive oil, sesame oil, virgin coconut oil.

Salt: Make the investment in a high-quality sea salt or Himalayan pink salt, a rock salt known for its superior mineral content.

Dried herbs and spices: Cocoa powder; vanilla powder; dried herbs and spices including black pepper, cardamom, cayenne, chipotle powder, cinnamon, cloves, cumin, garlic powder, nutmeg, onion powder, oregano, red chile flakes, thyme, turmeric, sage.

Flavoring ingredients: Apple cider vinegar, cacao nibs, capers, chickpea miso, sun-dried tomatoes, olives, truffle oil, vanilla powder.

Supplement(ary) Ingredients

Green powders: Spirulina and wheatgrass powders and other quality superfood supplements to green up your smoothies.

Protein powder: Make sure it's vegan and preferably not soy based; my favorite is Boku brand.

[62]

Vegan acidophilus powder: Probiotic powder (what you'd have if you emptied out an acidophilus capsule) used to make nut cheeses and yogurt; found in the refrigerated area of your natural food store's supplement section.

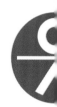

The Organic Avenue LOVE*Cleanses: LOVE*Easy, LOVE*Fast, LOVE*Deep, and Go Green

There's an Organic Avenue LOVE*Cleanse for everyone, whether you're testing the waters as a first-timer with **LOVE*Easy,** taking it a little further with **LOVE*Fast,** going all out with **LOVE*Deep,** or upping the alkalinity with **Go Green.** Organic Avenue doesn't subscribe to "one cleanse fits all," but all of our cleanse programs give your body a break from digesting heavy food, by infusing your system with pure plant-based nutrition and focusing the body's energy on healing. Our cleanses allow a release of the unLOVE*ing (detoxing) and increase the LOVE*ing (restoring): By including fruits and vegetable juices high in potassium, antioxidants, and chlorophyll, you'll remove acidity from the blood and tissues and thus restore alkalinity and balance to your whole system.

And guess what: You can eat while you cleanse! Organic Avenue's LOVE*Cleanses give you options with food and without, which is why we use the word *cleanse* rather than *fast*: Instead of evoking images of deprivation, cleansing becomes something all of us can do while maintaining our regular routines, going to work, exercising, and even dining out. Then, depending on your needs and interest, there are all-juice or all-green options to take cleansing to a more serious level and facilitate a deeper experience.

Flexibility is an important part of the Organic Avenue cleanses. Just as you would when ordering from the Organic Avenue boutiques, you can choose your number of days and your program, and if you need to change during the process, you are free to do so. You can mix and match the recipes as you plan the days of your cleanses and beyond. There are no steadfast rules here; this is an adaptable program capable of changing as your needs change. And they will change. That's part of the beauty of LOVE* and life. I do have one suggestion, though, to help ensure success: Plan ahead. Having the ingredients necessary and on hand will help you stick to your original plan and achieve your personal goals—and that will bring a greater sense of ease and satisfaction as you make it through this new experience. As you gain confidence with the recipes, you can begin to "wing it" and swap recipes with ease to accomplish the same goals.

Your Daily Cleanse Routine

We recommend making all your juices fresh for optimal nutrition; either make them just before drinking or make a day's worth in the morning, seal tightly, and refrigerate until you're ready to drink. If you have a grind and press juicer such as the Norwalk (see page 55), you can make juices up to three days in advance.

It's helpful to drink the juices and eat the foods in the order given, as they progress from lightest to heaviest throughout the day. This will help with digestion. If you are including fruit juice in your program, we like you to get that in first for optimal food combining. But if something isn't working for you, switch it up and experiment. See how it goes; if you notice indigestion or excess gas, switch back to the suggested routine.

WHY WE CLEANSE WITH GREENS (AND DON'T FAST ON WATER)

Greens are the staple of healthy detox, crucial to all of the LOVE*Cleanses. There's so much to love about the power of green: Greens contain first and foremost chlorophyll, which is the energy of the sun. Greens create healthy red blood cells and accelerate detoxification and rejuvenation. Greens also are the most nutritionally dense foods on a per-calorie basis, so when one is thinking about weight loss, healthy loss, it's vital to have low calories coupled with massive amounts of vitamins, minerals, and other nutrients. Enter green juices!

We could easily lose weight just drinking water, but without the nutrients that exist in green juices, a water fast could cause depletion and leave you hungry, and it wouldn't be sustainable. We want sustainable LOVE*! Green juices are so full of nutrition that you could easily consume as many of them as you can handle for days or weeks at a time. In fact, by going with the green you may actually be getting more nutrients by *not* eating than by eating!

[65]

LOVE*Easy (raw foods + juices)

LOVE*Easy is a gentle, complete introduction to living organic food: Think of it as Cleansing 101. It's a great starting point to acclimate your body to nutrient-dense, plant-based eating on the LOVE*Lifestyle. It's for people new to raw, living foods who don't practice a vegetarian or vegan diet or who have never cleansed before. Each day you'll be enjoying:

- A booster shot
- A fruit or carrot juice
- A vegetable juice
- A salad
- An entrée
- A dessert
- A mylk

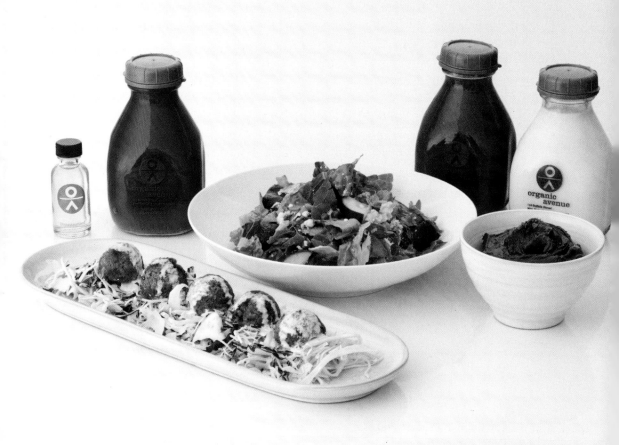

Most people think "juice" when they hear "cleanse," but raw foods are also cleansing thanks to their living enzymes and high water content. And an additional benefit of cleansing with foods is all the bulk and fiber vegetable foods provide, which work to keep the colon clean. LOVE*Easy teaches us how living foods can taste amazing without the guilt. The flavors are rich and super-satisfying, and you even get to eat dessert. There is no deprivation here!

LOVE*Easy is something we can return to when we haven't cleansed in a while. It's also a great option for times of stress or busyness when we're looking for the benefits of cleansing but need the support of nutrient-rich solids to bolster our strength and keep us going full speed.

If LOVE*Easy feels *too* easy, you can always change gears and switch out food items for juices, opting for the green variety as the best choice. Depending on your size and energy needs, LOVE*Easy can be seen as a food program. You can continue on it as long as you feel satisfied and you are losing weight or maintaining your weight goals. Everyone comes to cleansing from a different place, so the length of time is going to vary. As little as one day has its benefits, though a suggested five days works very well for most people as a good starting point. At the end of five days you can assess your goals and desires and consider going for another two to five days on LOVE*Easy or moving on to LOVE*Fast or LOVE*Deep. It's a very personal journey, and only you will know what you are ready to tackle. Ultimately your health is your responsibility, but a qualified health counselor, guide, or supportive friend can certainly help you stick with your plan and fully experience the LOVE*.

[67]

*LOVE*Easy Sample Menu*

1. Blue-Green Algae Booster Shot
2. Outstanding Orange Juice
3. Real LOVE* Green Juice
4. Kind Kale Salad
5. Happy Hummus Wrap
6. Cherished Chia Tapioca
7. Creative Cashew Mylk

LOVE*Easy Sample 7-Day Program

LOVE*Easy	Monday	Tuesday	Wednesday
Booster Shot	Cleansing Chlorophyll Booster Shot	Allowing Aloe Booster Shot	Blue-Green Algae Booster Shot
Fruit or Carrot Juice	Caring Carrot Juice	Precious Pear Juice	Outstanding Orange Juice
Vegetable Juice	Mighty LOVE* Green Juice	Smooth LOVE* Green Juice	Real LOVE* Green Juice
Salad	Kind Kale Salad	Big Greek Salad	Kind Kale Salad
Entrée	Thai Wrap	Fanciful Falafel	Lucky Lebanese Wrap
Dessert	Cherished Chia Tapioca	Cool Coconut Yogurt with fruit	Cherished Chia Tapioca
Mylk	Creative Cashew Mylk	Appealing Almond Mylk	Creative Cashew Mylk

[68]

Thursday	Friday	Saturday	Sunday
Wowing Wheatgrass Booster Shot	Allowing Aloe Booster Shot	Blue-Green Algae Booster Shot	Wowing Wheatgrass Booster Shot
Caring Carrot Juice	Gracious Grapefruit Juice	Wonderful Watermelon Juice	Clearly Coconut Water
Perfect LOVE* Green Juice	Smooth LOVE* Green Juice	Real LOVE* Green Juice	Mighty LOVE* Green Juice
Amazing Arugula Salad	Big Greek Salad	Kind Kale Salad	Amazing Arugula Salad
Thai Wrap	Fanciful Falafel	Magic Mushroom Wrap	Fanciful Falafel
Cool Coconut Yogurt	Cherished Chia Tapioca	Cool Coconut Yogurt	Cool Coconut Yogurt with fruit
Appealing Almond Mylk	Creative Cashew Mylk	Appealing Almond Mylk	Creative Cashew Mylk

LOVE*Fast (salad, soups, + juice)

LOVE*Fast is the second level of cleansing. It's a juice-based cleanse that includes a nice big salad at the end of the day. Reducing solid food intake speeds
up the detox process—without going too deep into an exhilarating liquid-only
regimen. Each day you'll be enjoying:

- A booster shot
- A fruit or carrot juice
- A tonic
- A green juice

- A soup
- A salad
- A mylk

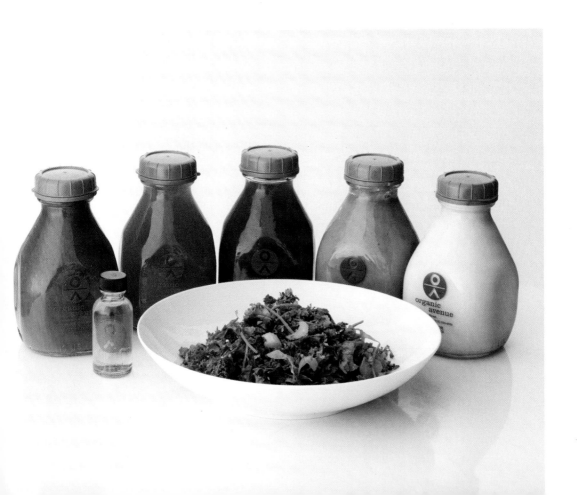

LOVE*Fast was Organic Avenue's first cleanse, launched in the early days. With the mostly juice program and the added benefit of fiber, you'll get the satisfaction of having all your nutritional cleansing goals met. For many people, including a substantial soup and salad makes all the difference; the solid food provides the sustenance and bulk needed for them to go the distance. LOVE*Fast is helpful for people who have the confidence that they are ready for less food and a more liquid experience. Again, a change can be made if you need more or feel you could do with less. Each day you will learn more about your body, its needs, and how well you are doing physically and emotionally. Many challenges encountered are not only physical; emotions that arise during a cleanse need releasing too. For some people, emotional release is a monthly event and crying is a common way to purge and release stuck emotions. Allowing for this emotional shift and realizing it is part of the process is important.

Choosing LOVE*Fast means things will happen more quickly. If you feel you are ready for that, go for it! If it seems too fast, you can slow the changes by switching to LOVE*Easy (page 65).

*LOVE*Fast Sample Menu*

1. Allowing Aloe Booster Shot
2. Precious Pear Juice
3. Truth Tonic
4. Real LOVE* Green Juice
5. Totally Tomato and Tarragon Soup
6. Big Kale Salad
7. Appealing Almond Mylk

LOVE*Fast Sample 7-Day Program

LOVE*Fast	Monday	Tuesday	Wednesday
Booster Shot	Cleansing Chlorophyll Booster Shot	Allowing Aloe Booster Shot	Blue-Green Algae Booster Shot
Fruit or Carrot Juice	Outstanding Orange Juice	Precious Pear Juice	Caring Carrot Juice
Tonic	Master Tonic	Truth Tonic	Generous Ginger Lemonade
Green Juice	Mighty LOVE* Green Juice	Real LOVE* Green Juice	Crazy LOVE* Juice
Soup	Terrific Tomato Basil Soup	Totally Tomato and Tarragon Soup	Terrific Tomato Basil Soup
Salad	Big Greek Salad	Kind Kale Salad	Amazing Arugula Salad
Mylk	Creative Cashew Mylk	Appealing Almond Mylk	Creative Cashew Mylk

[72]

Thursday	Friday	Saturday	Sunday
Wowing Wheatgrass Booster Shot	Allowing Aloe Booster Shot	Blue-Green Algae Booster Shot	Cleansing Chlorophyll Booster Shot
Caring Carrot Juice	Outstanding Orange Juice	Caring Carrot Juice	Clearly Coconut Water
Master Tonic	Truth Tonic	Generous Ginger Lemonade	Master Tonic
Smooth LOVE* Green Juice	Mighty LOVE* Green Juice	Real LOVE* Green Juice	Smooth LOVE* Green Juice
Totally Tomato and Tarragon Soup	Awesome Avocado Mint Soup	Totally Tomato and Tarragon Soup	Awesome Avocado Mint Soup
Big Greek Salad	Kind Kale Salad	Amazing Arugula Salad	Kind Kale Salad
Appealing Almond Mylk	Creative Cashew Mylk	Appealing Almond Mylk	Creative Cashew Mylk

[73]

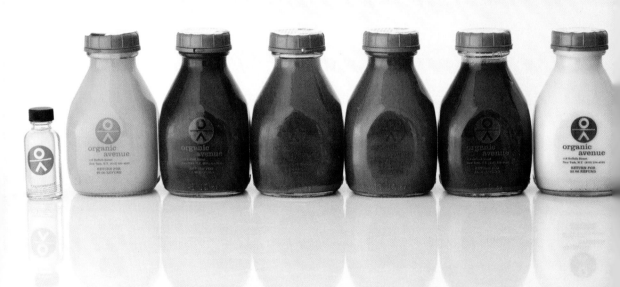

LOVE*Deep (all liquid nourishment)

LOVE*Deep is an all-juice cleanse with a mylk at the end of the day. It's great for veteran cleansers or those looking for the optimal mental and physical relief from preparing and digesting food. LOVE*Deep floods the body with pure hydration along with the highest quality nutrition available. When you give your body digestive rest, the many physiological repair mechanisms of the body have more energy to clean house. Each day you'll be enjoying:

- A booster shot
- A fruit or carrot juice
- Two green juices
- A vegetable juice
- A tonic
- A mylk

Nothing matches the surge of energy and clarity that comes from drenching the body with nothing but liquid nutrition, and the pounds will melt away in a most satisfying way. LOVE*Deep is just that, a deep dive into the cleansing process!

[75]

LOVE*Deep Sample Menu

1. Cleansing Chlorophyll Booster Shot
2. Outstanding Orange Juice
3. Smooth LOVE* Green Juice
4. Master Tonic
5. Cooling Cucumber Juice
6. Real LOVE* Green Juice
7. Creative Cashew Mylk

LOVE*Deep Sample 7-Day Program

LOVE*Deep	Monday	Tuesday	Wednesday
Booster Shot	Cleansing Chlorophyll Booster Shot	Allowing Aloe Booster Shot	Blue-Green Algae Booster Shot
Fruit or Carrot Juice	Gracious Grapefruit Juice	Caring Carrot Juice	Precious Pear Juice
Green Juice	Smooth LOVE* Green Juice	Crazy LOVE* Juice	Smooth LOVE* Green Juice
Tonic	Master Tonic	Truth Tonic	Grateful Green Lemonade
Vegetable Juice	Cooling Cucumber Juice	Caring Carrot Juice	Cooling Cucumber Juice
Green Juice	Real LOVE* Green Juice	Mighty LOVE* Green Juice	Real LOVE* Green Juice
Mylk	Creative Cashew Mylk	Appealing Almond Mylk	Creative Cashew Mylk

Thursday	Friday	Saturday	Sunday
Wowing Wheatgrass Booster Shot	Allowing Aloe Booster Shot	Blue-Green Algae Booster Shot	Cleansing Chlorophyll Booster Shot
Caring Carrot Juice	Clearly Coconut Water	Precious Pear Juice	Outstanding Orange Juice
Crazy LOVE* Juice	Smooth LOVE* Green Juice	Crazy LOVE* Juice	Smooth LOVE* Green Juice
Master Tonic	Truth Tonic	Generous Ginger Lemonade	Master Tonic
Caring Carrot Juice	Cooling Cucumber Juice	Caring Carrot Juice	Cooling Cucumber Juice
Smooth LOVE* Green Juice	Real LOVE* Green Juice	Smooth LOVE* Green Juice	Real LOVE* Green Juice
Appealing Almond Mylk	Creative Cashew Mylk	Appealing Almond Mylk	Creative Cashew Mylk

[77]

LOVE*DEEP: THE QUEEN OF ALL PROGRAMS

Though it's an advanced cleanse, just about anyone can dive into LOVE*Deep. (We recommend you consult your health-care provider before setting out.) This cleanse is designed to give you the greatest benefits in the shortest amount of time.

Most people are surprised to find the biggest challenge in going all liquid to be psychological willpower rather than physical yearning for food. Most report feeling satisfied on their cleanse, with happy bonuses of greater energy, less sleep needed, no midday slumps, increased clarity of mind, and a lift in mood.

Of course, if you have a caffeine or other addiction, the first couple of days may be a little up and down (see more about this on page 44), but if you trust and persevere, you will be pleasantly surprised, and before you know it you might find yourself saying, "I could do this forever!" You will begin to tell everyone how easy it is and how well you feel. And at around day five a newfound confidence in the power of plant-based nutrition most likely will appear. And don't be surprised if next time you decide to take it a step further and opt for a low-sugar, super-high-alkaline Go Green cleanse for an even deeper experience. You are sure to learn more about yourself each step of the way.

Go Green

Go Green is a low-glycemic-index version of LOVE*Deep; it simplifies the options and steps up the alkalinity with a menu consisting of all-green chlorophyll-rich juices and soups. It's for our experienced cleansers who seek to keep on prevention's good side, or those in a health crisis or who have maxed out on the SAD (standard American diet) and are looking to call in the reinforcements.

Each day you'll be enjoying:

- A booster shot
- Crazy LOVE* Juice
- Three green juices
- A tonic
- A mylk

Go Green Sample Menu

1. Cleansing Chlorophyll Booster Shot
2. Crazy LOVE* Juice
3. Smooth LOVE* Green Juice
4. Grateful Green Lemonade
5. Real LOVE* Green Juice
6. Smooth LOVE* Green Juice
7. Clearly Coconut Mylk

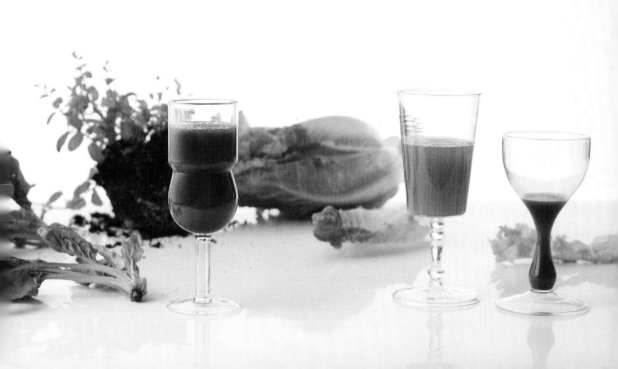

Go Green Sample 7-Day Program

Go Green	Monday	Tuesday	Wednesday
Booster Shot	Cleansing Chlorophyll Booster Shot	Wowing Wheatgrass Booster Shot	Blue-Green Algae Booster Shot
Crazy LOVE* Juice	Crazy LOVE* Juice	Crazy LOVE* Juice	Crazy LOVE* Juice
Green Juice	Smooth LOVE* Green Juice	Real LOVE* Green Juice	Smooth LOVE* Green Juice
Tonic	Grateful Green Lemonade	Master Tonic	Grateful Green Lemonade
Green Juice	Real LOVE* Green Juice	Smooth LOVE* Green Juice	Real LOVE* Green Juice
Green Juice	Mellow LOVE* Juice	Real LOVE* Green Juice	Smooth LOVE* Green Juice
Mylk	Creamy Coconut Mylk	Appealing Almond Mylk	Creative Cashew Mylk

[80]

Thursday	Friday	Saturday	Sunday
Cleansing Chlorophyll Booster Shot	Wowing Wheatgrass Booster Shot	Blue-Green Algae Booster Shot	Cleansing Chlorophyll Booster Shot
Crazy LOVE* Juice	Crazy LOVE* Juice	Crazy LOVE* Juice	Crazy LOVE* Juice
Real LOVE* Green Juice	Smooth LOVE* Green Juice	Real LOVE* Green Juice	Smooth LOVE* Green Juice
Master Tonic	Generous Ginger Lemonade	Truth Tonic	Truth Tonic
Smooth LOVE* Green Juice	Real LOVE* Green Juice	Smooth LOVE* Green Juice	Real LOVE* Green Juice
Real LOVE* Green Juice	Smooth LOVE* Green Juice	Real LOVE* Green Juice	Smooth LOVE* Green Juice
Appealing Almond Mylk	Creative Cashew Mylk	Creamy Coconut Mylk	Appealing Almond Mylk

Choosing Your Cleanse

	LOVE*Easy	LOVE*Fast	LOVE*Deep	Go Green
Who's it for?	First-timers, those who haven't cleansed in a while, and anyone looking for a food-containing cleanse	Those ready for a second level of cleansing, while keeping a little solid food in the program	Those looking to take their cleanse to a high level, to jump in and do some serious cleaning house	Experienced cleansers, those maxed out on SAD, and those looking to up the green in their cleanse
What's included?	Fresh juices and living foods	Fresh juices, soups, and salads	Fresh juices	Green juices and soups
Why do it?	To get the benefits of juices plus the colon-cleansing fiber of living foods	To speed up the detox process without going full-force into a liquid-only program	To give yourself the benefits of pure liquid nutrition in the shortest amount of time	To step up the alkalinity and take your cleanse deeper than deep

Hydrate for Health

Ever feel hungry, then drink a glass of water and the hunger's gone? Sometimes when we think we're hungry we're really just thirsty. That piece of knowledge might clue you in to the importance of staying hydrated.

The body is composed of at least 65 percent water, and water is a major component of the blood, so staying hydrated means you are keeping the blood healthy and clean. Purified water and the pure water of plants in the form of fresh juices are excellent hydration choices.

Dehydration is linked with all sorts of chronic disease, pain issues, and fuzzy thinking. Our ability to recognize thirst diminishes as we age, and many elders admitted to the hospital for various reasons are actually found to be dehydrated. Even early labor signs can point toward dehydration, not to mention how many athletes end up on drips after letting their precious fluids sweat out before replacing them.

Think of staying hydrated as a lifelong project, which, with all the tonics, juices, mylks, and other forms of hydration that are part of the LOVE*Lifestyle, shouldn't be too difficult to accomplish!

[83]

Adding water to your day is easiest when you begin first thing in the A.M. with a tall glass, perhaps with a squeeze of lemon to jump-start your digestion. Then you'll be hydrating all day as you enter the LOVE*, cleansing and enjoying the array of liquid recipes you'll find in the pages that follow.

Getting quality water requires some planning. Even if your city takes pride in its municipal water, you might think twice before drinking it straight from the tap. Consider this: Only 91 contaminants are regulated by the Safe Drinking Water Act, yet more than 60,000 chemicals are used in the United States according to the Environmental Protection Agency. The Safe Drinking Water Act was passed in 1974—it's more than thirty years old. Not a single chemical has been added to the list since 2000. It's time for an update!

Alkalinity is important, so the more we can boost alkalinity from the water and juice we drink and the food we eat, and by reducing unnecessary stress in our life (everything from polluted air to polluted relationships), the better. Utilizing an alkaline water machine or supplementing with bottled alkaline water (as we do at Organic Avenue) can help, and a few super-simple sneaky tricks like adding a little sodium bicarbonate (baking soda) to your water can help too. Helpful travel hint: Take a bottle of pH drops (see Food and Equipment Sources, page 317) with you in your bag. Dropping these liquid magicians into your water will raise that alkalinity and even purify a host of parasites, bacteria, and other unseen and unwanted travel companions.

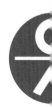

Releasing the unLOVE*ing, aka Toxins, During Your Cleanse

As you transition to the LOVE*Lifestyle and diet, symptoms of detoxification through cleansing are to be expected. When you cleanse, the process of detoxing from the unLOVE*ing can speed up considerably, and you may feel worse before you feel better. The length of the cleansing process depends on the diet you've favored going into your cleanse: If you are making a drastic switch, your symptoms may be strong; if you have avoided the use of caffeine, nicotine, sugar, and alcohol in the past, your detoxification symptoms may be quite mild or nonexistent. (See more on detox from these substances on pages 44 to 45.)

Just so you know, some possible detox symptoms include flatulence, skin eruptions, increased thirst, cravings, runny nose, headaches, irritability, constipation, insomnia, nervousness, coated tongue, fatigue, aches and pains, weakness, diarrhea, edema, nausea, cold and flu symptoms, bad breath, frequent urination, and loss of appetite. Now, don't be scared off: Some of us get some of these symptoms, but not everyone gets all of them. And the good news is that detox symptoms are a sign that your body is becoming healthier each day as the body rids itself of accumulated waste. If you feel overwhelmed by symptoms, consider slowing the detox down. Add some steamed veggies, and that should do it. And you can help the process of cleansing along by engaging in some or all of these unLOVE*ing-releasing practices.

Releasing the unLOVE*ing Through the Skin

We all feel great after a good soak in the tub or a spell in a sauna. Perhaps it's because these practices help to bring out and release unLOVE*ing through the skin, which happens to be the largest organ of elimination. Think acid management instead of asset management! Our skin is often a guide to the health of our other organs, and acne and other skin eruptions can be the result of toxic or overworked kidneys and liver and a stagnant colon. All of these organs will use the skin to expel the unLOVE*ing if they cannot process them quickly enough. How to get the unLOVE*ing moving out of your system through the skin during your cleanse? Here are a few delightful ways.

- **Dry skin brushing:** Before your morning shower, brush all over the body in a clockwise circle for a natural gentle exfoliation that is at once invigorating and relaxing. Dry skin brushes are available at many natural food stores and shops that sell products for the bath.
- **Epsom salt baths:** Pour 1 to 2 cups of Epsom salts in hot water and relax in the bath for about 20 minutes; as you do so, the salts will work to draw unLOVE*ing out of your body through your skin. Add a few drops of essential oil for a relaxing spa experience.
- **Sauna:** Take a 10- to 45-minute sauna with cold shower breaks in between (this also helps the circulatory system). Infrared saunas are particularly valuable in releasing unLOVE*ing, especially heavy metals, through the skin. And it's a great opportunity for self-massage!

Releasing the unLOVE*ing Through the Lymph

Our bodies also can release toxins through the lymphatic system. To facilitate this process, there are several practices you can engage in during your cleanse. Hydrotherapy is especially recommended if the body is not eliminating regularly during your program. After all, it's not a cleanse unless the toxins leave your body!

- **Dry skin brushing:** In addition to detoxing through the skin (see opposite), dry skin brushing stimulates the lymphatic system.
- **Exercise:** I recommend low- or no-impact activities like rebounding, yoga, walking, swimming, stretching, and breathing exercises to keep the system moving. An easy walk will gently encourage lymphatic circulation; a sweaty workout will push unLOVE*ing out more quickly. Really listen to what your body needs. On LOVE*Easy, our food-based program, most people can exercise comfortably. If you're on LOVE*Deep or another extended juice-only regime, be mindful to not overexert. Sometimes rest can be the greatest purifier. And sweating via hot baths and/or saunas will encourage purging of those pesky poisons.
- **Massage:** Deep-tissue, lymphatic drainage, and Thai massage are all beneficial during your cleanse in your efforts to flush out toxins. And they are a treat that you deserve for embarking on this cleansing journey. A natural facial, body scrub, or herbal body wrap would be an added bonus. Remember to drink plenty of fluids before and after in order to effectively flush away anything unLOVE*ing that's been stirred up.
- **Colon hydrotherapy:** Engaging in colonic treatments is a great way to assist the body in removing toxic waste. See Deepening Your Cleanse with Enemas and Colonics on the following pages for more on your options.

[87]

DEEPENING YOUR CLEANSE WITH ENEMAS AND COLONICS

In the interest of taking your cleanse to a deeper, colon-cleansing level, let's put modesty aside for a moment and consider the benefits of enemas and colonics. When we eat a live-food diet or are fasting, the high enzymatic content contained in these foods is stirring up old waste matter that has been impacted in the colon. With an enema or a colonic, we are using water to flush the system: Think of it as an internal bath. This practice, very Old World, is just resurfacing in the United States.

A few health conditions can make colon cleansing dangerous, so always check with your doctor to see if enemas and colonics are right for you. Generally, though, they are very safe and very beneficial: By assisting you in a more complete elimination, removing excess buildup of waste, enemas and colonics help to purge toxins from the colon. Colon cleansing can also relieve constipation, something that can happen when you're on an all-juice cleanse. Other benefits of colon cleansing may include strengthened immunity, clearer skin, and weight loss, and an even more efficient colon as it gets cleansed, toned, and strengthened.

Should you go for an enema or a colonic? It depends on your budget and the level of cleansing you're after. You may want to consider your living structure: Some may find it easier to go to a hydrotherapist to keep the process more private; others may want to educate and learn hygienic practices together as a family. Some may sneer at first but will be thanking you later. Don't let others deter you from becoming empowered to take control of your health.

Enema: An enema works to cleanse the lower part of the colon via a single infusion of water; it can be done yourself with a kit bought from a pharmacy following the instructions included. It's a highly affordable at-home colon-cleansing method. An enema bag can be your best travel companion. Most people who travel know that constipation is a frequent unwanted result, usually stemming from dehydration and poor food choices or lack of bathroom access. You can reboot your system by utilizing an enema bag, and this way you can continue your healthful LOVE*Lifestyle or cleanse while on the road.

Colonic: A colonic, or colon hydrotherapy, is always done by a professional colon hydrotherapist in her office: It does the work of an enema and more by cleaning the entire length of the colon and removing impacted waste from the large intestine via multiple infusions of water into the colon. Colons that have suffered the standard American diet are usually inefficient at elimination, and the extra cleaning really helps. If your budget and time allow for it, it's worth trying it out for the extra cleansing effects. Experienced colon hydrotherapists are usually knowledgeable about the LOVE* Lifestyle and diet and can give you the encouragement you need during your cleansing experience. Always look for a qualified, certified practitioner, ask about their water filtration system, and get some referrals. Do your homework and meet with the therapist beforehand.

Colema Board: A Colema Board is a third option, a cross between an enema and a colonic, and something you can do yourself at home. It's potentially more thorough than an enema, as it works to give a complete cleansing to the lower colon. Buying one involves an initial investment of $300 or so, but it's a one-time expenditure and something you might consider as you strengthen your commitment to cleansing.

[89]

Releasing the unLOVE*ing Through the Emotions

We hold emotions in the body, and in every cell we hold memory. The liver holds anger, the kidneys hold fear, the gallbladder holds frustration. When we cleanse, these emotions have the opportunity to be released. The body is an amazing miracle, and is always headed toward healing. These cleansing symptoms are all signs that our body is releasing unwanted debris and emotion that has accumulated over the years. Even though it can be uncomfortable, I urge you to embrace the miracle that this is nature doing its finest healing work. Here are a few suggestions on how to work to a place of emotional expansiveness and freedom.

- **Meditate:** Starting or continuing with a meditation practice works to clear the mind and center yourself (see more on meditation on pages 34 to 37). Clarity of mind and heightened awareness are common side benefits of cleansing, so cleansing can be an ideal time to deepen your meditation practice.
- **Practice the power of positive affirmations:** Here's one that works for me: "Every minute that I cleanse I am flushing more unLOVE*ing from my system. Every hour that I cleanse I become healthier and have more energy and youthfulness."
- **Rest and relax:** It is very important to allow both your physical and emotional body to rejuvenate during this process. Something as simple as lighting a candle during your evening bath or before bed can provide nurturance.

[90]

> 📖 *Catch yourself thinking. Meditation gives you a great clue to how fast you are really moving. You may be sitting still yet exhausting yourself with your thoughts, as your body can experience your thoughts quite literally. Learn to let go of thoughts . . . watch them . . . do not attach to them."*
> —DENISE MARI

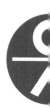

The LOVE*Cleanse FAQ

Q: *How long should I cleanse, and how often?*

A: It is completely up to you. To experience good results, we find that five days are optimal. However, you will be doing some good work even if you can only do one day of juicing and live vegan foods. Many people like to cleanse seasonally, but some will do a cleanse once a year or once a month. The most important part is maintenance, incorporating live foods into your daily diet, creating healthy habits, choosing mostly alkaline foods, and reducing your unLOVE*ing intake, and then cleaning house with our specific cleanse programs from time to time. You can try each cleanse program from LOVE*Easy through LOVE*Deep for three weeks for a total of twenty-one days. I promise you will feel amazing. We recommend working closely with a health counselor who can guide you to make realistic goals for yourself and help you monitor your progress. Remember, on a LOVE*Cleanse you are not fasting or starving; rather, you are cleansing and eating and drinking in a healthful way. And cleansing is not just about weight; it's about being healthy, making periodic cleansing important whether or not you have weight to lose.

Q: *I don't have much time, but I'd like to cleanse. Is it useful to do a cleanse for just one day?*

A: Absolutely! One day can be very helpful. For some, a brief cleanse can be a confidence-building exercise that leads to more intensive cleanses. Others might add one day a week ongoing. It's always good to add more fresh, ripe, raw, organic, plant-based food and juices, and if you have only twenty-four hours for a cleanse, you'll still reap the benefits.

Q: Is there any reason I shouldn't start out with an all-liquid cleanse? Can I detox too quickly?

A: Cleansing should not be a race to the finish line. You don't score more points if you jump in to LOVE*Deep on your first cleanse. In fact, you might have a more successful cleanse if you do LOVE*Easy (which includes solid food) on your first one. The fiber in solid food requires more digestive work, thus slowing down the detox process. This is okay; it allows your body to get rid of the toxins your cells release at a steady pace. If you dump too many toxins at once, your body will not be able to remove them quickly enough and they will only be reabsorbed (this is a retox).

Picture a shelf that has accumulated an inch of dust; it is not really a problem right now. This is equal to stored gross toxins in your cells. Now take a feather duster and dust the shelf. All of the dust is now in the air, causing you to cough and sneeze. Alkaline green juices are the feather duster awakening the toxins. The coughing and sneezing are the uncomfortable detox symptoms. Now the actual cleanse part is removing the dust from the air; in our bodies, this means eliminating. Eliminating happens when we breathe, sweat, and move our bowels. It is essential to make this happen when cleansing to avoid re-toxing (before the dust just settles on the shelf again). See the suggestions on pages 85 to 90 to help keep the toxins moving along. If you are experiencing severe symptoms, see a doctor.

Q: What about juicing only until dinner? I have business dinners that I need to attend, and I don't want to seem antisocial.

A: Many of us long-term juicers frequently "stay liquid" until dinner. Just make sure you drink enough so that when you sit down for dinner your hunger doesn't cause you to overeat. Most restaurants will accommodate special diets. You can ask for a good bottled water, a nice vegan soup, and a hefty salad. Ask with a smile and you'll likely get a lovely, healthy meal that might even inspire your colleagues to do their own cleanse!

Q: *Is an alkaline cleanse the most effective kind?*
A: Yes! The short answer: Disease thrives in an acidic system; health reigns in a slightly alkaline one. The longer answer: Eating a plant-based diet, drinking pure water, living a lower-stress life, and breathing clean air helps the body become alkaline. (See more on alkalinity on pages 11 to 12.) But much of the stuff of the standard American lifestyle and diet—including animal protein, dairy, coffee, soda, alcohol, sugar, environmental pollutants, and stress—creates acid in the body. Our bodies do their best to maintain balance in this external and internal onslaught of acid. However, if we become too acidic, a tipping point occurs, and excess acidity is thrown into the tissues to preserve the pH balance of the blood. At this point, our bodies begin to break down, with our weakest areas affected first. According to some nutrition experts, most diseases are caused by the blood becoming too acidic. An alkaline cleanse is the only kind that will help balance your pH level and allow you to thrive from a cellular level.

[93]

Q: *I'm nervous about cleansing. I don't want to feel sick, deprived, or out of my element. What should I do?*
A: We totally feel you! Trying new things can cause anxiety. Thoughts of so-called failure can be overwhelming. The good news is there's nothing to prove! You can try out a cleanse, and if you feel like you need more food, you can have it. If you crave something else and it's a healthy food, you can have it. If something feels off and you want to stop, you can. Every little step counts toward your overall health. And each little bit of cleansing adds to your health. Even if you do only one day, or even half a day, it's a great start. You're creating a

new food foundation for yourself—a more nurturing, nutritious, and loving way of being with food. And as you continue to cleanse, you may find it gets easier each time and you may feel more comfortable extending the amount of time you cleanse. Check out our online community and Cleanse Concierge Service for support at any stage of the cleansing process. Find a buddy. Whether online or in real time, having a friend begin the process with you can really help.

Q: When should I not do a cleanse?

A: Listen to your body. If you feel junked up, tired, fatigued, and achy, and have a lot of blemishes, gas, or any other symptoms of unwellness (consult your M.D. if you feel it's serious), consider resting and increasing your water intake first. But if you feel your normal self (even if your normal self is a tad run-down), go for a cleanse. If you feel that you want to eat solid food, you can always go easy with LOVE*Easy. A cleanse should feel right to you—don't allow yourself to be pressured into it. Do not cleanse if you are pregnant or breast-feeding. Unless you are already a full-fledged LOVE*r, switching your diet drastically when pregnant or breast-feeding is not a good idea. Increasing healthy goodness is great, of course, but if you're carrying a new life or caring for a newborn, make those changes gradually.

Q: How much weight will I lose on a cleanse?

A: Every body is different. If you're already slim and eating well, you may not lose any weight at all. Others who are overweight and transitioning from a highly processed, low-nutrient diet may lose a pound a day. Losing weight can be tricky for some who have been heavy their whole lives and easier for those who've gained rapidly over a shorter period of time. But all is possible, and remember to keep positive during the process. We see our programs as the beginning of a lifestyle shift to eating more nourishing, nutrient-dense, plant-based foods. If you continue the delight of discovering these and learning more, the weight you shed should stay off. We also think it's more supportive of yourself to ask "How healthy and alkaline will I be?" or "How much will I glow?" To us, the answers to those questions rather than "How much weight did I lose?" are how we measure the success of our programs. LOVE* yourself for where you are and who you are, and allow love to fill yourself during the process. No matter what the weight-loss result, know that you are treating yourself the best you can, and that is all that truly matters.

Q: *How can I keep the weight off after I have finished my cleanse?*
A: Like any learning process, the more you immerse yourself in the beginning, the stronger your foundation will be. That means understanding intellectually why you're eating this way, and experientially understanding it too. Once you know what to eat to calm your cravings and how to keep your body's systems optimally functioning, you'll be free to make great, nourishing food choices for the rest of your life. There will be less of a focus on weight and more of a focus on finding the optimal you. Don't compare yourself to others, be kind to yourself, and enjoy the process.

[95]

Q: *Will I feel hungry during my cleanse?*
A: Probably not. It depends on the cleanse program you choose and how much you usually eat. On LOVE*Easy there's so much to consume you may not finish it all. On a liquid cleanse like LOVE*Deep you may be hungry initially, but the hunger should quickly go away. Drinking water between nutritional beverages helps keep the hunger at bay. If your hunger doesn't pass and you feel like you may give in to a "cheat," choose a living food like a salad, avocado, or fresh fruit so you can stay the course. And if you do "cheat," I've got news for you: There are no rules. Just say OK, I will do a little better tomorrow; no self-flagellation allowed. And who says feeling hungry is necessarily so bad? Now that I have been cleansing for many years, when I feel hungry I feel progress. I know my body is going to go to work on something other than digesting. If losing a little weight was the goal, then welcome a little hunger. These are short-term cleanse

programs that deliver powerful nutrition during the process, so if a hunger pang happens along, notice it and let it go. It, too, will pass.

Remember to go to sleep relatively early, 9 to 10 P.M. Often if one stays up too late (11 and beyond), hunger will show up and tempt you in the wee hours. Don't risk the temptation during a cleanse; rest instead. Get the most of this time you've dedicated to your healing process.

Q: What about watching calories?
A: Some of our pure plant juices have a high calorie content (calorie counts are available on the Organic Avenue website). This can be a little alarming to a calorie-counting mind-set. But we value high nutritional content and quality ingredients over calories, something we consider an outdated system of food measurement. According to some experts, counting calories is born from a perspective that sees the stomach as a furnace that requires energy to burn an element to ash. Thanks to the alkalinity pioneers, we think of the stomach as an alkalinity contributor. People gain weight when they're consuming the meat and potatoes of the SAD (standard American diet)—or even the sugary fruits and processed wheat and oils in many vegetarian, even vegan, diets. People stay slim when consuming fresh vegetables and low-sugar fruits. We suggest dropping the calorie conversation and focusing on the ingredients themselves. Are they whole foods, plant-based, raw, organic, and alkaline? If yes, eat to your heart's delight. Yet be mindful that if your diet is full of animal products, wheat, and processed foods and you add a smoothie on top of that, yes, you'll be overconsuming. So think about allowing our delicious, high-nutrient recipes to replace your standard vittles and see how satisfied—yet not overfull—you'll feel. And just drop the math.

Q: What are the benefits of the green juices compared to fruit juices?
A: We believe that the chlorophyll in green plants, leaves, stems, and grasses gives the body all it needs to make healthy blood. And that's the first step in

creating a healthy body. Green juices contribute alkaline minerals. Although fruit contains natural sugar in the form of fructose, all sugar—even fructose—is acidic and potentially damaging, tapping the body's reserves, often leaving lower pH environments and putrefying in the gut when consumed in excess. But the cleaner your system gets, the more you'll find yourself drawn to leafy greens and green fruits like cucumber and avocado that can be consumed liberally. A little fruit juice goes a long way; drinking fruit juices diluted is a good idea, especially for children and those with sugar sensitivity. Though when you're new to the LOVE*, enjoying a fruit feast can be a good introduction. Think of it like birthday cake: You wouldn't have it every day, but a slice once in a while makes life just that much sweeter.

Q: I can't get the green juices down; I've tried everything—is it okay if I just skip them?

A: Some people really struggle with the greens at first—but it's worth it to keep trying. Check out our varied options—it's possible you just don't like one of the ingredients: Real LOVE* Green Juice contains pear and lemon to help it go down; Mighty LOVE* Green Juice has easy-to-drink cucumber; Smooth LOVE* Green Juice is a little more of a serious green; Cooling Cucumber Juice is extra-easy and great for beginners. You can also try adding apple (preferably a green apple), carrot, or lemon—generally, this helps the green medicine go down. If you've tried them all and still have challenges . . . go find a straw, hold your nose, and *just drink it*! Kidding. Sort of. But really, see if you can stretch your-self. It's very likely that as your body absorbs the nutrients and feels how great that is, you'll eventually develop a taste for them. If you are really having a strong reaction to the greens, ease into them super-slowly with baby steps. Just don't give up on the greens—they are truly lifesavers.

[97]

Q: Should I continue to take my multivitamins during a cleanse?
A: It's up to you. Some people have no problem taking vitamins as usual, but some supplements are too strong to be taken on a juice-only stomach without food as a buffer. If you're ready for a multivitamin break, during your cleanse would be a good time.

Q: What should I do if my stool is bloody?
A: First, take a closer look—is that blood or is that beet juice? If the water is tinged pink and there's no blood on your body, then it's probably beet juice. Beets will also dye your urine a bit, so see if that's the case too. If so, no worries! If it is blood, it could be hemorrhoids or fissure caused by constipation or something more serious. It's wise to consult your doctor. And then continue toward a fiber- and nutrient-rich Organic Avenue approach to balance and heal.

Q: I haven't moved my bowels at all since I started my program. What should I do?
A: It's uncomfortable but not unusual. The bowel can slow when on a juice-only program. So we suggest keeping things moving with 2 to 4 ounces of aloe (see page 110) twice a day (this often works wonders and can also help with any nausea you may feel). Enemas, colonics, or a Colema Board (see page 89) can work magic for moving the bowels.

Q: Why is it important to eliminate during a cleanse?
A: It's actually essential to eliminate at least once a day. Moving your bowels two or three times a day is recommended, yet most of us do not. The uncomfortable fact is that some people are carrying up to eighteen meals in their gut! We believe bowel challenges are at the root of most health problems. Some wellness experts say that if you mess with this fundamental bodily system (as our standard American diets do), then you mess with your ability to produce healthy blood, absorb nutrients and water, and eliminate waste.

Q: *Can I cleanse while I'm pregnant?*

A: You and your growing baby will thrive on a nourishing variety of whole, organic, clean, fresh food. But pregnancy is not the time to make extreme changes, detox, or diet. So if you're currently eating a high percentage of processed foods, refined flours, sugars, and meat, consider a gentle shift—adding fresh fruits and veggies (especially greens), pure juices, nuts, seeds, seaweeds, and more to the mix. Our Creamy Coconut Mylk (page 189) is a favorite of pregnant women; they find it helps them maintain energy and gives them that "yum" feeling they crave. As much as you want to do the right thing and eat healthfully when you find out you are preggers, don't overdo it. Don't kick-start the cleansing process now. You are eating for two, and more is required when you are pregnant.

Q: *Is it safe to cleanse while breast-feeding?*

A: See above—most of the same principles apply to pregnancy and breast-feeding: Make no radical shifts, check with your doctor, and be sure to get plenty of nourishment, including many fresh foods and juices in your diet. In case this isn't clear enough: No cleansing when breast-feeding! No radical shifts. Gradual is OK, because who doesn't want to give their growing baby the very best? But, I repeat, no radical changes during breast-feeding. And eat, as you are going to need the extra energy to keep your body healthy while providing the nourishment to grow a baby.

[99]

Q: *Can I cleanse if I have diabetes?*

A: Absolutely—many have controlled or eliminated type 2 diabetes through a living foods diet. But definitely consult with your doctor first. Then, with her support, consider the LOVE*Easy cleanse if you'd like the convenience of a program. And consider switching some of the fruit juices for the Go Green options. If you can't find an M.D. who is confident in this direction, consider checking the Resources section (page 307) for health retreats; many have walked the path before you, and if you can get yourself into the right hands, you may just surprise your physician, family, and friends. Again, this is not a radical program, but a calculated, educated, informed, intentional change with experienced support.

Q: *Can I do the cleanses if I am lactose or gluten intolerant?*
A: Absolutely! There are no animal products or by-products in any of our recipes. The recipes are wheat- and gluten-free as well. Yay!

Q: *Is there a cleanse for candida issues?*
A: Yes—try Go Green. All of our cleanses address cleaning the colon, which is where candida thrives. Once that is clean and restored to balance, candida no longer has a home in your body—but beneficial, healthy bacteria do. The perspective that I picked up while studying with alkalizing guru Dr. Robert O. Young is that an acidic environment contributes to the breakdown of cells, and yeast is a natural by-product of this breakdown. In turn, it's a nasty process of recycling, but if you're not dead, there is no need to compost your body. Clean it up instead and bathe the cells with alkalinity so the breakdown stops and a healthy balanced body is the result.

Q: *Can I smoke on the cleanse?*
A: Though we can empathize with all kinds of addictions, it's ideal to stub out the smokes while you cleanse. Many smokers use their cleanse as an opportunity to quit. They often find that once their system is supported by the optimal nutrition a raw, plant-based diet provides, their cravings subside. You'll be amazed to see what naturally, easefully falls away during even a brief five-day break from toxic substances. If you really need a boost to kick the butts, take a peek online at some pictures of people with emphysema. I know firsthand, as my grandfather, bless his soul, died from it, and it is one of the worst ways to go.

Q: Can I cleanse while taking antibiotics or other medications?

A: It's best to check with your M.D. if you're taking any medications. Especially be mindful of the grapefruit juice while on some medications. With some medications you can't even have greens! You will need to check with your doctor and get serious about eliminating the cause that has led to a pharma-toxic dependency, especially one that dictates no fresh fruits and veggies or their juices.

Q: Can I cleanse if I have a cold?

A: Definitely. At the first sign of any cold symptom, first look at what you have been eating, then at how your bowels are functioning (are they moving two or three times a day?). If the answers are not pretty, you can start juicing, reducing solid food intake, engaging in bowel cleansing via colonics, and sweating via a sauna or hot baths. Add proper rest, and no more cold—works for us every time. Though if your symptoms last more than a week or so, consult your doctor.

Q: What age is suitable for cleansing? When is too young?

A: You're never too young to start eating well! But obviously kids need to ease into any change, and they don't need to cleanse like adults, even if they have acquired grown-up food addictions and weight issues (childhood obesity has more than tripled in the past thirty years, a sobering fact). Check with your child's doctor and proceed slowly, making changes fun and preparing food together. This is a chance for a lifetime shift—there's no rush, and it's a learning opportunity for you both. You could start by adding some new live plant foods and alkaline water. Keep quantities plentiful, provide variety, and make sure kids have foods that offer comfort, nurturing, and great taste. Let the loving connection between you—"Vitamin L"—be the largest ingredient while you're trying new healthful foods. Also find community with other families and children eating a wholesome LOVE*-based diet.

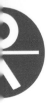

Transitioning Back After Your Cleanse: Maintaining What You've Attained

Whether you nourished yourself gently with LOVE*Easy, sped the detox with LOVE*Fast, or drenched your cells with LOVE*Deep, it is an accomplishment to be fully acknowledged. Your body has been waiting all its life for such complete nourishment. Since an unadulterated, live food, organic, and vegan diet is other than the norm for most people, generally there is a transitional period of detox and adjustment. Some feel basically great all the way through, others have slight digestive disturbances and other mild symptoms, and still others have more intense detox symptoms as the body recalibrates to the higher level of nutritional vibrancy. This transition can be a challenge and it can also be fun—and the LOVE* does not have to end. Continue to treat yourself with utmost honor and respect: Choose to break your cleansing program gently.

Prepare your home for the day after your cleanse with fresh fruit and salad ingredients. When you awake, drink fresh water to hydrate yourself, followed by a fresh green vegetable juice. Next, have your fruit of choice, chewing conscientiously (we recommend choosing fruit in season). When you're hungry again (preferably a few hours later), enjoy a big green salad. If you participated in the LOVE*Deep program, omit adding beans, grains, and dense protein sources to your salad on this day. You can, however, add avocado if you like. A wonderful dinner choice is a simple green salad topped with steamed veggies.

The consumption of whole, plant-based nutrition during your cleanse should be a practice carried with you throughout your life, at whatever level works best for you. As you reincorporate grains and legumes into your modified LOVE* diet, do so slowly. Pay attention to how you feel. I believe that there is no biological need for animal flesh, and I recommend keeping it out of your diet. If you are craving dairy and eggs, choose organic, or better yet, check the Food and Equipment Sources section on page 317—I will show you what I eat to replace those animal foods for good. It takes a little while to retrain yourself; over time new foods replace the old and the cravings will be for more healthful, more life-affirming foods. Be patient, be aware, and watch as cravings shift and new habits are formed.

Be sure to reach for fresh green juice and raw salads long after your cleanse is over. Who knows, you may be inspired to do another one next week!

The recipes in this book make it easy for you to continue to incorporate fresh-pressed juices, living meals, desserts, and snacks into your life. Eating organic raw fruits, vegetables, and other plant-based foods is a lifestyle choice of abundance. It is entirely accessible to anyone committed to feeling great. Our recipes offer you the framework to ease you into this vibrant lifestyle and to support you as you prepare your meals.

[103]

The recipes, which you'll soon be getting to, can also be used as a transition *into* a cleanse. Again, no hard-and-fast rules, just the pure pleasure of eating and drinking your way into a healthy body.

As I've mentioned, the LOVE*Lifestyle is not all or nothing, and that goes for the incorporation of consciously cooked vegan foods. Eating some cooked foods doesn't necessarily mean you eat only cooked food: That would be a significant detour from healthy habits. So if you find that happening, jump on another LOVE*Cleanse so you can remember how good you feel when you consume pure living food full of energy and vibration. If you decide to introduce one consciously cooked meal per day, the final meal of the day is a good choice, because the energy requirements for metabolizing cooked food are very real, and you are better off having that "slump" in the evening as you are heading toward relaxation, meditation, and bed—rather than when you are waking up and looking toward utilizing all your energy for your creative endeavors, whether work or play (of course you could add a cooked element like a grain, baked sweet potato, or other vegan choice as an accent to any raw meal). On the other hand, a lazy Sunday brunch could also be a good time if rest and relaxation are your goals and your energy needs aren't a high priority (yet be prepared for a nap if you do!). You know your lifestyle and energy requirements best, and now you have the food of LOVE* tools at hand to guide you.

> ❝ *There are mysterious forces making sure we get what we need in this lifetime. If you ask, you will receive. Prepare yourself to receive!"*
>
> —DENISE MARI

A Typical LOVE* Day, Post-Cleanse

My morning routine is easy: I feel a sense of satisfaction starting my day with a smoothie, generally a green smoothie, especially in the spring and summer months, or when I am boosting the LOVE* in my life. There are infinite variations of green smoothies one could make (see pages 171 to 177 for the Organic Avenue recipes). A green smoothie repertoire is a breakfast problem-solver for all ages. Get this happening first and you are sure to start off on the best foot regardless of what comes next. Green smoothies can be tweaked toward low-glycemic or high protein or both! It's really a blended salad, when it comes down to it. They are fast to make, cleanup is minimal, they are easy to take on the go, and they are quick to consume. I know this is something we all can appreciate when running for the door but wanting to make sure we are fully nourished before we launch into our day.

Lunch is a great time to keep up the raw routine. Think soup and salad, choosing from the blended soups that you can drink if you're on the run and hearty full-of-fiber salads that will give you what you need, especially if topped with avocado, olive oil, lemon, and sea salt. If you feel that you need more, enjoy larger portions or consider adding snacks such as hummus with crudités or a few nuts to get you to dinner.

Dinner can be a repeat of lunch, with even more emphasis on green and veggie protein, such as one of our wraps (pages 241 to 249) or zucchini or other pasta options (pages 258 to 267). If you're eating out, look toward the healthful veggie side dishes, adding avocado to salads, requesting olive oil for steamed veggies with a sprinkle of sea salt, or indulging in the restaurant vegan entrées that are thankfully becoming more and more commonplace. Add fruit for dessert, or enjoy a macaroon, some chocolate mousse, or any of the other Organic Avenue desserts (see pages 279 to 298) to end your LOVE*-filled day. Now let's head over to the kitchen for the LOVE*Recipes!

[105]

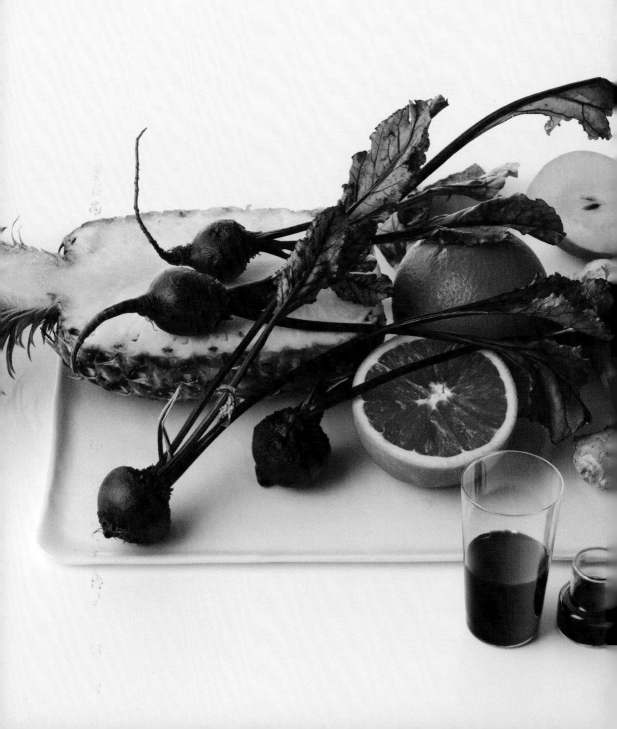

PART III

The LOVE* Potions: DIY Booster Shots, Vegetable and Fruit Juices, Tonics, Smoothies, and Mylks

The LOVE* potions are liquid magic. They form the backbone of the LOVE*Cleanses and they support you daily as part of your Live. Organic. Vegan. Experience. **Booster shots** are compact, concentrated energy sources—from aloe to wheatgrass—that you can use as a quick pick-me-up or add to any drink to boost the nutrition. **Vegetable and fruit juices** are powerful in their simplicity, loaded with vitamins, minerals, and other nutrients. **Tonics** are light, water-based drinks generously flavored with turmeric, ginger, lemon, and other healing ingredients. **Smoothies and mylks** are blended nuts, fruits, and veggies in a glass, full of fiber and whole food nutrients. Try them all, mix and match ingredients, and drink your way to radiant health and a LOVE*-filled life.

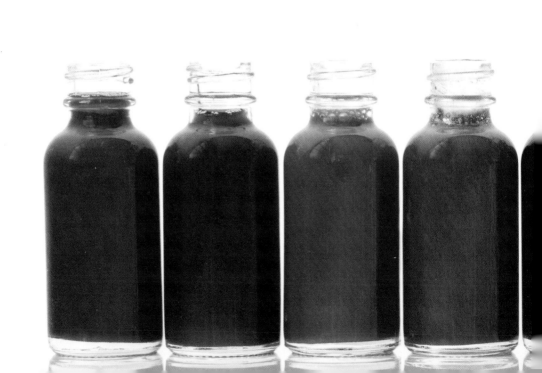

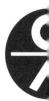

Booster Shots

Booster shots are concentrated health and energy delivery systems; taken in little one-ounce amounts, they give a dose of fun but lifesaving liquid minerals, vitamins, and aminos. They can be sipped alone or added to water, juices, smoothies, mylks—any of the Organic Avenue liquid offerings—as a daily supplement or as a quick pick-me-up when energy is at a lull. If you're drinking your boosters straight up, serve them in shot glasses, or find yourself a bunch of one-ounce glass bottles and do as we do at the Organic Avenue boutiques and divide them into portable, pocketbook-size individual servings.

[109]

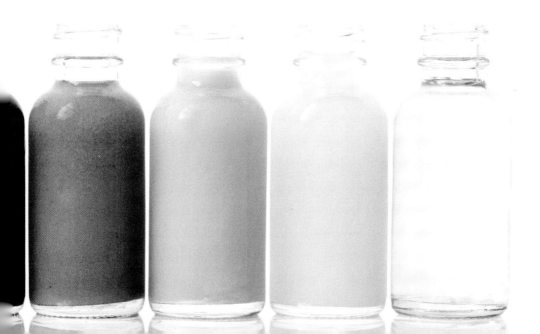

Allowing Aloe Booster Shot

Made from the plump stalks of the succulent aloe plant, Allowing Aloe can help detoxify the body, from the colon to the bloodstream. It is also calming to the stomach and entire digestive tract. You can find a quality brand of aloe vera juice at your local natural food store or online, or get down to it and make your own by following these steps:

1. Find yourself a healthy aloe plant and pull off a leaf.
2. Take a sharp knife and peel the rind from the leaf and discard.
3. Remove the yellow layer just under the rind to reveal the aloe gel. For every 2 tablespoons gel you remove, you'll add 1 cup (240 milliliters) water.
4. Place the aloe and water in the blender and blend until smooth. Drink it straight up or mix it with additional water or juice; it goes particularly well with strong citrus flavors.

Lovable Lemon Booster Shot

Refreshing, cheery, and uplifting, a shot of pure lemon is one great way to start the day. Or mix it with a glass of water and the vegan sweetener of your choice and you have a glass of good old-fashioned lemonade. Lemon soothes a sore throat, eases indigestion and constipation, cleanses the stomach, and boosts immunity. Have some on hand to finish soups, to mix with oil and herbs for salad dressing, or to add spark to any recipe that needs a little extra something. To make your stash of lemon juice, just peel as many lemons as you like and run them through the juicer, or, alternatively, juice them by hand with a citrus reamer.

Power Pom Shot

Who needs red wine when pomegranate juice will give you even more anti-oxidants, with bonus heart-protective, anti-inflammatory, and anticancer effects? Cut open as many pomegranates as you'd like (you'll need about 5 pomegranates for 1 cup of juice—no wonder bottles of this crimson elixir are so pricey!), scoop out the seeds, and run them through your juicer. Combine with another fruit juice, dilute with water, or take a private moment to slowly savor it solo.

Ginger Gem Booster Shot

We LOVE* ginger, can't say enough about it. It's nature's miracle root, soothing upset stomachs, relieving bloating and gas, and enhancing assimilation of food and nutrients. This anti-inflammatory, antioxidant-rich immune booster is a must-have, one to keep a generous supply of in your refrigerator's crisper drawer to make multiple boosters. To do so, simply run a bunch of knobs of ginger through your juicer, or for small amounts try using a dedicated ceramic ginger grater or a completely clean garlic press. Drink straight up for a hit of warming relief from a cold, or mix it with a smoothie, juice, or seltzer and a little vegan sweetener of your choice for a real-deal ginger ale.

[111]

Cleansing Chlorophyll Booster Shot

Whether you drink it as is or mix it with water or another drink, this booster is all about regeneration and cleansing at both the molecular and cellular levels. Chlorophyll is known to help fight infection, neutralize bad breath, heal wounds, and keep your circulatory, digestive, immune, and detoxification systems in working order. Chlorophyll also increases red blood cell count, thereby improving how your body absorbs and uses oxygen. Who couldn't use a nice hit of O_2 every now and again? Find a quality brand in a bottle at your natural food store or online and fill your glass up often! Don't fret if it colors your teeth chlorophyll green; just swish some water in your mouth and the green will be gone.

Blue-Green Algae Booster Shot

Blue-green algae is a gift from the ocean to LOVE*. It gives you an astonishing blast of concentrated vitamins, minerals, and enzymes. It's a must on the LOVE*Lifestyle. It's a powerful immune and brain booster, good for the digestive system, and a mood stabilizer. It also increases oxygen uptake, making it a wonderful workout companion. Our favorite is E3 Live online (see Food and Equipment Sources, page 317).

Wowing Wheatgrass Booster Shot

According to Dr. Robert O. Young, author of *The pH Miracle,* and other health experts, the chlorophyll molecule in wheatgrass is almost identical to the hemoglobin molecule in human blood. The theory is that chlorophyll can then transform into hemoglobin, increasing red blood cell count and the body's capacity to deliver oxygen to the cells of the body. Wow! Get your wheatgrass any way you can—freshly made from your local natural food store or, if you're a DIY person, invest in a dedicated wheatgrass juicer (see Food and Equipment Sources, page 317), grow your own grass, and make yours fresh from your kitchen windowsill garden. Most wheatgrass will be gluten-free, as long as it is *pure* wheatgrass—just the grass, not the seeds, which contain gluten. Be sure to check your sources.

BIG PROPS TO THE MOTHER OF WHEATGRASS, ANN WIGMORE— AND HER GRANDMOTHER

Ann Wigmore, who founded the Hippocrates Health Institute (now called the Ann Wigmore Institute, located in Puerto Rico) in 1968, was the first to introduce wheatgrass as the cornerstone of a living foods diet. But the mother of wheatgrass would never have earned that title without her grandmother.

Ann Wigmore was born in Lithuania in 1909 and was raised by her self-taught naturalist grandmother. This heroic woman saved the lives of many wounded World War I soldiers on both sides by feeding them and treating their wounds with herbs, weeds, and grasses under conditions of great peril.

After Ann immigrated to the United States as a teenager, an automobile accident shattered her legs. Gangrene set in, and doctors recommended amputation. Ann refused, intuitively feeling there was a better way. She remembered the healing power of grasses she learned about from her grandmother and returned to a diet of vegetables, grains, seeds, and greens. She picked wild weeds and greens and applied them to her feet, and she ate as many greens as she could. Her bones fully healed without surgery (and she later went on to run the Boston Marathon).

In the 1950s Ann called on her grandmother's green wisdom again to heal herself of colon cancer. Ann went on to develop a health and healing system based on a live foods diet with an emphasis on wheatgrass that has benefited many lives at the Ann Wigmore Institute. "Living foods for living bodies, dead foods for dead bodies," is how the mother of wheatgrass put it.

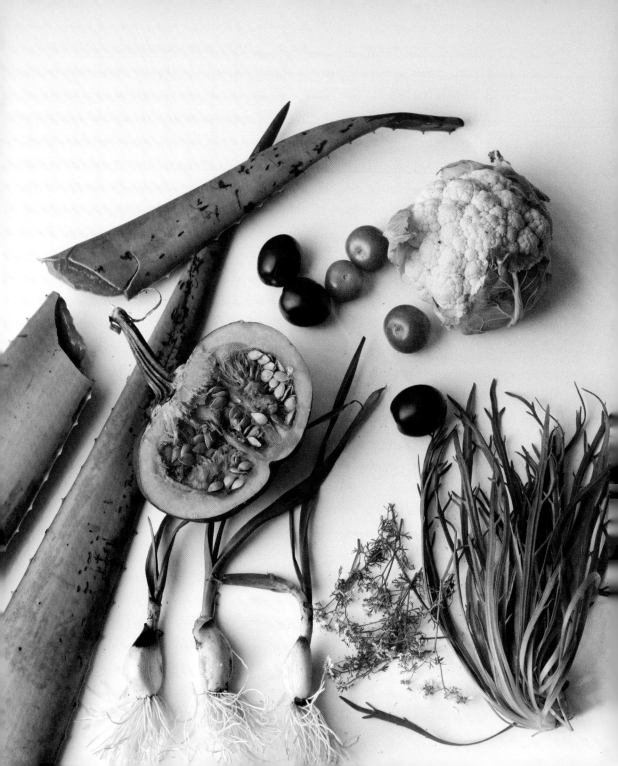

Vegetable Juices

Vegetable juices are the heart and soul of the LOVE*Cleanses and an important part of the everyday LOVE*Lifestyle. Vegetable juices are both delicious and nutrient dense, full of vitamins, minerals, and chlorophyll; they immediately flood your cells with hydration and nutrition without requiring a lot of energy to digest them. So kick back with a tall one and relax, knowing you're giving your system a rest while you're drinking up. And did you know that many green drinks contain close to or the entire RDA of veggies? Don't stop there! Go, LOVE*, go!

A few things to keep in mind when you're juicing:

- Your juices will taste a bit different each time because thanks to the miracle of nature, no two vegetables are exactly the same.
- Your yield will vary too, based on the size, juiciness, and ripeness of your produce and the type of juicer you use. If you use a grind and press juicer such as the Norwalk, your yields may be a bit higher than those given in the recipes.
- Juice the ingredients more or less in the order given in the recipes; start with small items like ginger and lemon, and finish with larger, juicier vegetables like cucumbers to avoid having small bits of small ingredients remaining in the juicer at the end.
- To increase the yield, run the pulp through the machine once after all the veggies have gone through.
- Include the stems from your leafy greens—they are completely juiceable. You can save the stems from your collard and kale salads to add to your juicer as well.
- Favor seasonal and local vegetables when you can.
- Remember this bit of advice if you are green shy: You can acclimate your palate to greens—the more you favor green, the easier it is to eat and drink those greens in copious quantities.

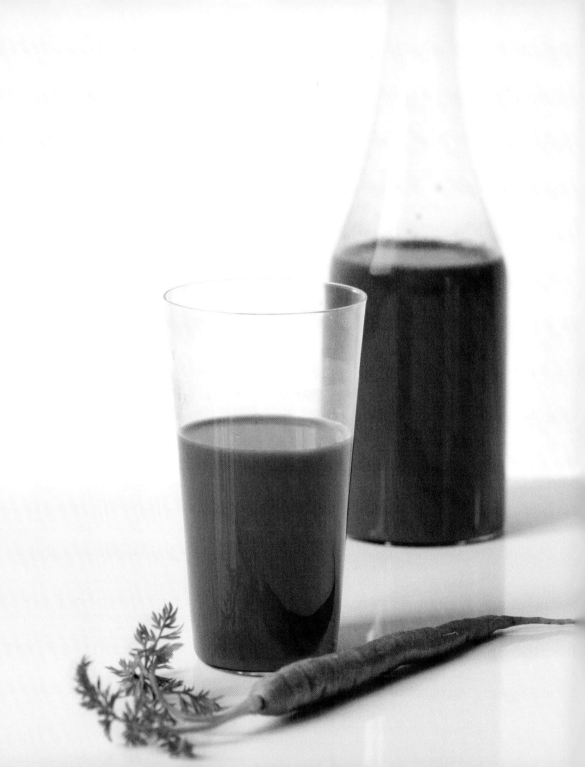

Caring Carrot Juice

Kids love it for its sweetness, adults are fond of it for its versatility; you really can't go wrong with carrot juice! The carrot is the original juicing vegetable. It's often used as a base for mixed juices or to add a hit of vegetable sweetness to any juice, something good to know for folks who are new to juicing greens. In fact, some say it's the carrot juice that's responsible for that characteristic "live food glow" often found radiating from those following the lifestyle. My three-year-old son, Oliver, has been thriving on carrot juice, watered down for his young little system.

And that truism about carrots helping you see better? My friend Joel Seiden will attest to it; after implementing a high-carrot-juice regimen, at age sixty-two, he no longer needs his glasses. It may have something to do with the carrot's super-high vision-supporting vitamin A content (vitamin A deficiency can lead to night blindness, a widespread condition in developing countries).

> **NOTE**
> No need to compost your pulp; save it to make Organic Avenue's very own Caring Carrot Cheese (page 220).

Makes about 16 ounces (470 milliliters)

2 pounds carrots, scrubbed and ends trimmed (about 12 medium carrots)

Run the carrots through a juicer, pour into glasses, and serve, over ice if you like, or pour into a container, cover, and keep in the refrigerator until ready to serve.

> **DID YOU KNOW?**
> You need to scrub carrots to get a bright and glistening orange-colored carrot juice; if you simply wash those carrots, your juice may wind up a muddy brownish color. So invest in a two-dollar brush and give your carrots a thorough cleaning before they go through the juicer.

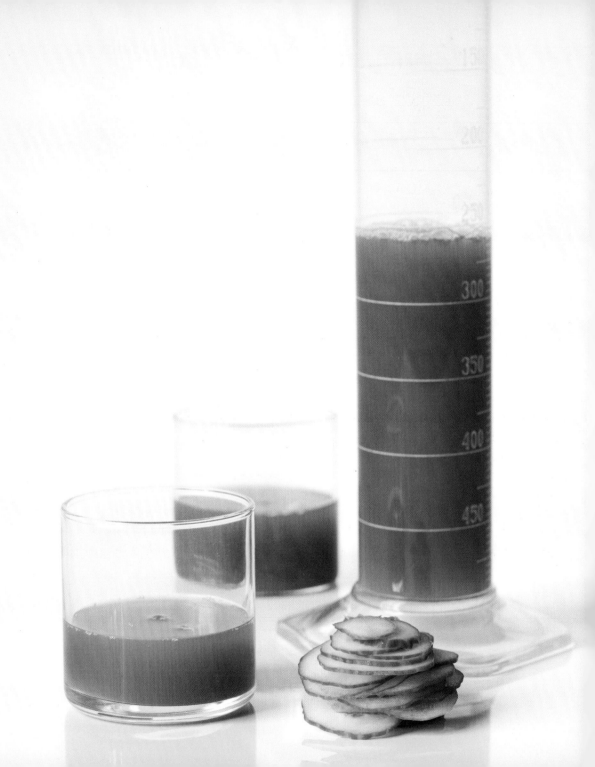

Cooling Cucumber Juice

Refreshing and a pretty shade of green, Cooling Cucumber is an icebreaker for people new to drinking green, and the one I tend to grab in the summer and drink like water. Cucumbers are low glycemic, anti-inflammatory, and rich in antioxidants including vitamin C and manganese. Cucumbers also contain a phytonutrient called cucurbitacins that is the subject of exciting research regarding their anticancer properties, something to watch out for as more information is revealed.

Makes about 16 ounces (470 milliliters)

2 large unpeeled cucumbers (about 1½ pounds/680 grams), ends trimmed and
   roughly chopped

Run the cucumbers through a juicer, pour into glasses, and serve, over ice if you like, or pour into a container, cover, and keep in the refrigerator until ready to serve.

[119]

LIKE A SPA IN A GLASS
Though it's cooling, cucumber juice is also calming and hydrating, like a spa in a glass. To further your spa experience, apply the cucumber pulp to your face to make a face mask; relax with it for about 30 minutes before washing it off. And don't forget to save a couple of slices to place over your eyelids for that extra bit of indulgence.

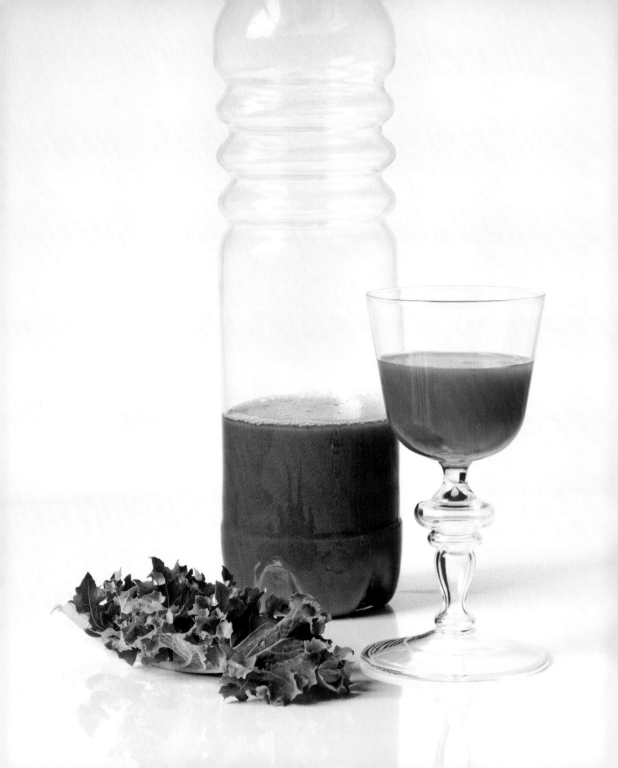

Real LOVE* Green Juice

This was my first veggie juice love, from back in the early days when I was experimenting with going green. Real LOVE* is surprisingly smooth: The dark leafy greens, heavy on the kale, are balanced by hydrating cucumber; pear provides sweetness and body, and lemon adds a lightness and brings the flavors together.

Makes about 14 ounces (420 milliliters)

½ lemon, peeled
½ pear, stemmed and roughly chopped
½ cup (20 grams) roughly chopped cilantro leaves and stems
4 kale leaves, including stems
4 romaine lettuce leaves
1 Swiss chard leaf, including stem
3 celery stalks, with leaves
1 unpeeled cucumber, ends trimmed and roughly chopped

Run all the ingredients through a juicer. Pour into glasses and serve, over ice if you like, or pour into a container, cover, and keep in the refrigerator until ready to serve.

[121]

DID YOU KNOW?

Unlike most greens, kale takes on more flavor and color after the weather turns cold. It withstands and even thrives in the frost of late fall and winter, when greens season is long past in most parts of the country. So dedicate a large garden plot to kale to keep a steady supply going or search out winter farmers' markets to keep the locavore spirit going all through the year.

TARGETED DRINKING

If you're looking to up your intake of a certain vitamin—say, vitamin A to improve or maintain your vision—pull out the juicer and drink those vitamins! Juicing delivers a potent, targeted vitamin punch. For example, an 8-ounce glass of carrot juice will give you as much as 35,000 IUs of vitamin A (about 800 percent of the RDA), in the pure form of beta carotene, which is easily converted to usable vitamin A in the liver. (Synthetic vitamin A can be toxic in large doses; see more about the hazards of synthetic vitamins on page 29.) You can drink your vitamin B complex with green juices and sprout juices; drink your vitamin E with beet, celery, and green juices; and drink your vitamin C with just about any fresh fruit and vegetable juice. And the minerals in juices are also easy to assimilate; a diet high in fresh juices ensures that you are getting the minerals you need.

If you're looking to ease a certain condition, pull out the juicer again (or better yet, make dedicated counter space for your juicer). Specific juices can target any number of conditions: Peptic ulcers can be treated with cabbage juice, prune juice has a laxative function, watermelon and cucumber juice act as diuretics, and those beautiful orange, yellow, and green colors that get even more concentrated in a cup of fresh vegetable juice are being closely looked at as potential preventives for certain cancers.

From anemia to infections, liver disorders to lung disorders, menstrual problems to sinus disorders . . . you name it, there's a plant or juice of a plant that can be helpful. The pharmaceutical industries are on it—and creating synthetic versions of these potent plant extracts. Consider skipping those pills, pulling out the juicer, and getting ahead of any potentially preventable diagnosis the natural way. Start juicing for the LOVE* of it!

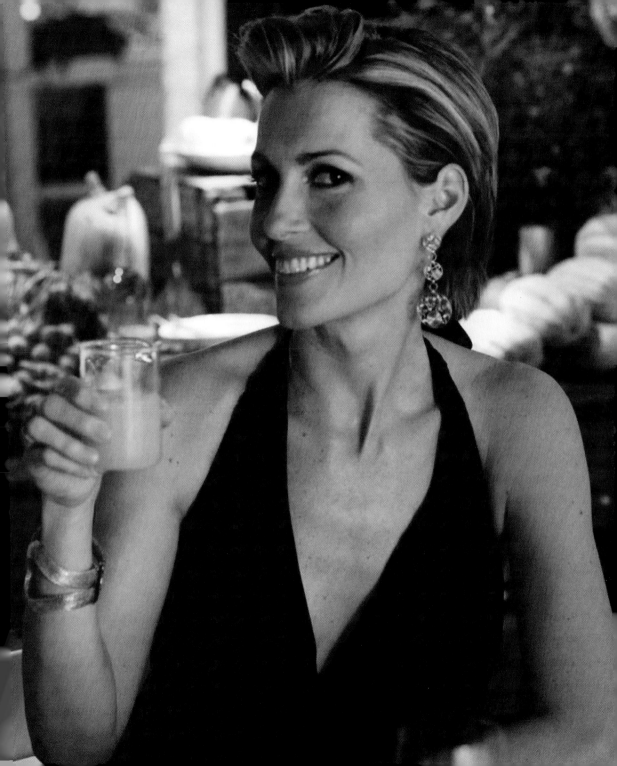

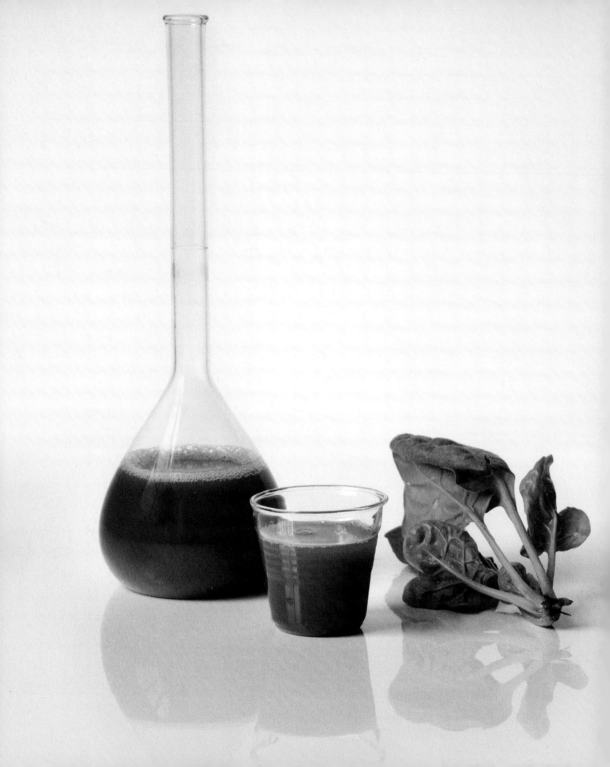

Smooth LOVE* Green Juice

If you are looking for a straight green juice, without fruit or another sweetener, but something smooth, not too bitter, this drink is the answer: With mild-mannered cucumber and romaine lettuce offsetting deeply green spinach, Smooth LOVE* becomes an oft-repeated recipe.

Makes about 14 ounces (420 milliliters)

1 unpeeled cucumber, ends trimmed and roughly chopped
2 celery stalks, with leaves
5 romaine lettuce leaves
1 Swiss chard leaf, including stem
1 cup (30 grams) roughly chopped parsley leaves and stems

Run all the ingredients through a juicer. Pour into glasses and serve, over ice if you like, or pour into a container, cover, and keep in the refrigerator until ready to serve.

> **DID YOU KNOW?**
> Some people report feeling a little nauseated when they first add green juices to their diet. This could simply be because you are detoxifying quickly, so good going! But you may want to start slowly in the beginning, build up to all-green juices, and add a Ginger Gem Booster to your greens to offset that unsettling feeling.

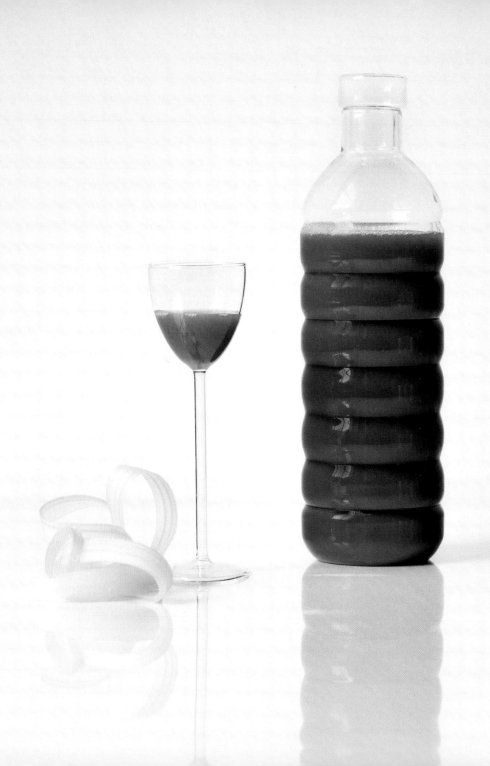

Mighty LOVE* Green Juice

Light and easy, a celery and cucumber base with a small amount of kale or collards makes this a perfect green drink for newbies and a super-hydrating summer staple.

Makes about 14 ounces (420 milliliters)

4 medium celery stalks, with leaves
1 large unpeeled cucumber, ends trimmed and roughly chopped
1 kale or collard green leaf, including stem

Run all the ingredients through a juicer. Pour into glasses and serve, over ice if you like, or pour into a container, cover, and keep in the refrigerator until ready to use.

DID YOU KNOW?
While most people think of the cucumber as a vegetable, it is in fact a closet *fruit,* in the same botanical family as melons. Which may explain why, if you close your eyes, cucumber juice on its own could be mistaken for watermelon juice.

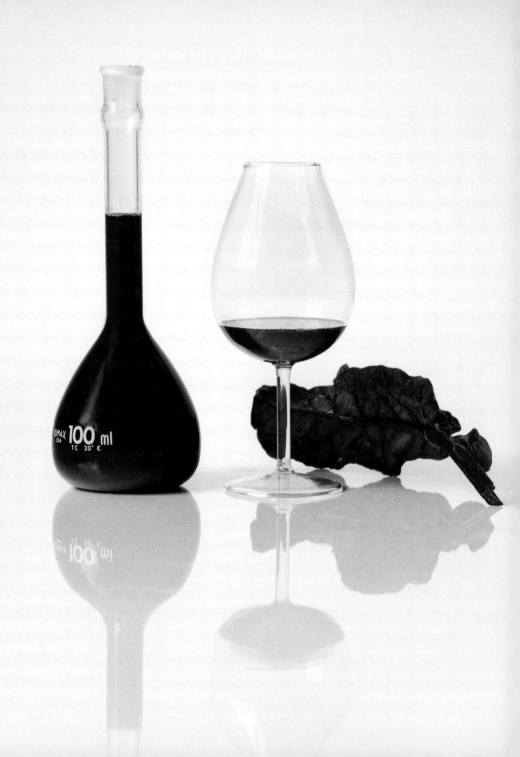

Perfect LOVE* Green Juice

Let's get in touch with our roots: carrots and beets, which you'll find in just the right amounts to provide natural sweetness, in perfect balance with green leafy vegetables and a touch of lemon to finish.

Makes about 14 ounces (420 milliliters)

½ lemon, peeled
½ cup (20 grams) roughly chopped cilantro leaves and stems
1 kale leaf, including stem
Handful of spinach leaves
1 carrot, scrubbed and ends trimmed
½ large beet, scrubbed and ends trimmed
3 celery stalks, with leaves
½ unpeeled cucumber, end trimmed and roughly chopped

Run all the ingredients through a juicer. Pour into glasses and serve, over ice if you like, or pour into a container, cover, and keep in the refrigerator until ready to serve.

[129]

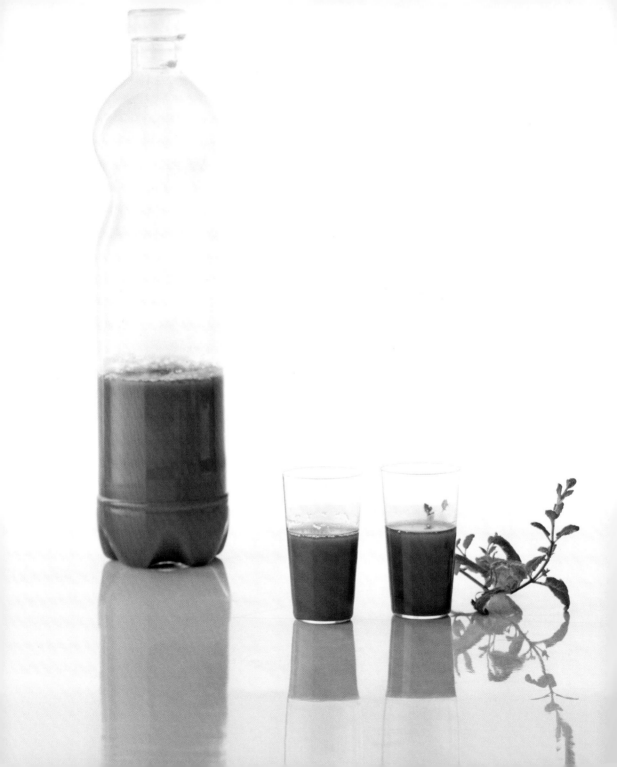

Grand LOVE* Green Juice with Garlic

This green juice, with its generous amounts of medicinal dark greens and garlic juice, is magically healing and fiercely detoxifying—enough to keep the vampires away and the sniffles at bay. It contains more vitamin A, C, and E than exists in most four-course meals, with no cholesterol and negligible amounts of fat. Turmeric adds anti-inflammatory effects. Try it as a nutrient-dense, low-calorie meal replacement when you're cleansing.

Makes about 14 ounces (420 milliliters)

½ lemon, peeled
½-inch (1.25-centimeter) piece fresh turmeric
1 garlic clove
4 collard green leaves, including stems
2 handfuls of spinach leaves
1½ unpeeled cucumbers, ends trimmed and roughly chopped
Small pinch of cayenne
Pinch of salt

[131]

Run the lemon, turmeric, garlic, collard greens, spinach, and cucumbers through a juicer. Stir in the cayenne and salt. Pour into glasses and serve, over ice if you like, or pour into a container, cover, and keep in the refrigerator until ready to serve.

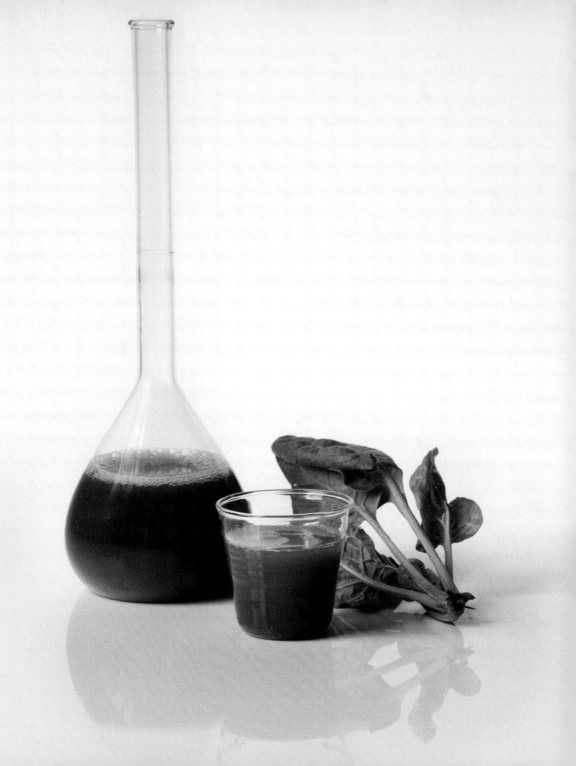

Sweet LOVE* Green Juice

Here the flavor of the fruit overshadows the intensity of the greens and makes it perfectly palatable for even the most anti–green food eater!

Makes about 14 ounces (420 milliliters)

1 medium pear, stemmed and cut into quarters
2 collard green leaves, including stems
2 kale leaves, including stems
1 Swiss chard leaf, including stem
Handful of cilantro, including stems
½ unpeeled cucumber, end trimmed and roughly chopped
½ lemon, peeled
2 oranges, peeled and quartered

Run all the ingredients through a juicer. Pour into glasses and serve, over ice if you like, or pour into a container, cover, and keep in the refrigerator until ready to serve.

[133]

DID YOU KNOW?

Some, but not all, pears contain iron. How do you know? If your pear turns brown when you cut it, it contains iron; if it doesn't, it has little or no iron. Pears also are a good source of vitamin C, which is an iron enhancer, so the vitamin C in the pears helps you absorb and maximize the iron already found in the pears. Nice teamwork!

Super Green Juice

Very green but mild because of the cucumber, this juice has a bit of lemon for a nice contrast. If you've got a bunch of one of the greens but none of the others, feel free to substitute, mix, and match as you wish—you'll never go wrong by going green, whatever the combination.

Makes about 14 ounces (420 milliliters)

1½ large unpeeled cucumbers, ends trimmed and roughly chopped
1 collard green leaf, including stem
1 kale leaf, including stem
1 Swiss chard leaf, including stem
Handful of spinach leaves
½ lemon, peeled
½ bunch cilantro, including stems
½ small bunch parsley, including stems

Run all the ingredients through a juicer. Pour into glasses and serve, over ice if you like, or pour into a container, cover, and keep in the refrigerator until ready to use.

TIP
If you're shy about juicing leafy green vegetables, try adding a booster of chlorophyll to a glass of Cooling Cucumber Juice (page 119) to get more green into your system. Chlorophyll has a pretty neutral taste and for the most part disappears in the cucumber.

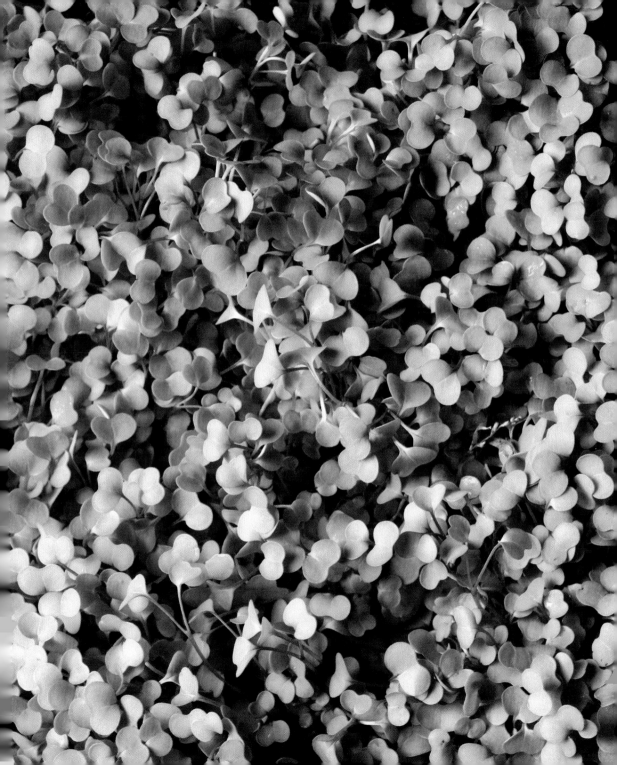

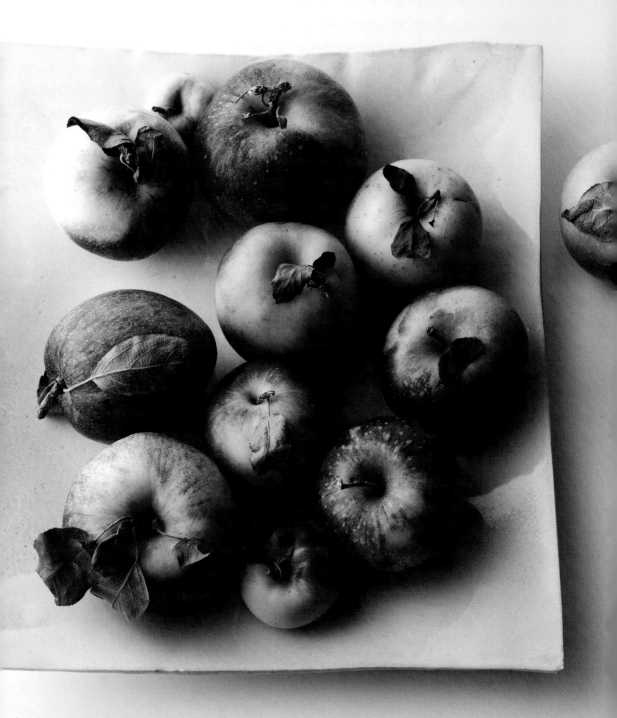

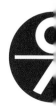

Fruit Juices

You'll need no convincing of the deliciousness of the Organic Avenue fruit juice repertoire: Whether it's everyone's favorite orange, perfectly bitter grapefruit, or clear and lightly sweet coconut, the fruit speaks for itself. As with the vegetable juices, no two fruit juices will taste the same; it all depends on the season, the size of fruit, its level of juiciness, and the type of juicer you use. Here are some additional tips:

- Favor seasonal fruits when you can for the most delicious results, and avoid any fruits with blemishes or bruises: Quality into the juicer, quality out!
- Go ahead and dilute any juice with water if you find it too sweet, and start your kids off with juices that are about 80 percent diluted.
- Introduce a wide range of flavors early to children so they can develop a wider palette and LOVE* freely as they grow.
- Mix and match your fruits to come up with your own signature combinations—this is where you can get really creative in the kitchen!

[137]

Once you make a commitment to juicing, be it with vegetables or fruits or both, you'll see how simple and delicious the process is. After all, you are (literally) squeezing more nutrition and life force into your body, becoming empowered as you take your life, your health, and your family's health into your hands.

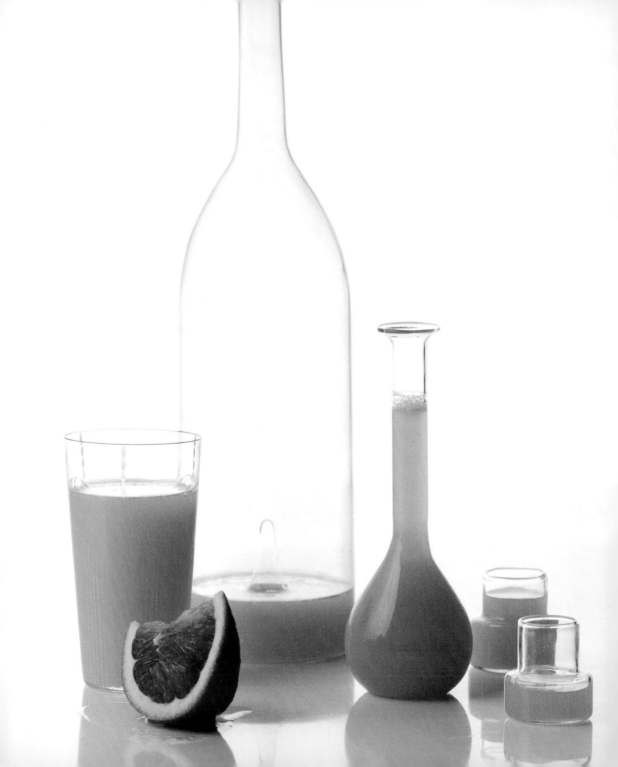

Outstanding Orange Juice

There's nothing like fresh orange juice. Pasteurization kills nutrients and kills flavor. I've never met a woman, man, or child who didn't love a fresh glass of OJ! And one orange has more than 100 percent of the U.S. RDA of vitamin C; drink a tall glass of orange juice and you'll be several times ahead of the game. It pays to stick to the real thing: A University of Milan study found that vitamin C–fortified drinks and vitamin supplements don't give the same benefits as drinking orange juice. And juicing your oranges soon after opening them ensures that you're getting the most benefits, as oranges start to oxidize and lose vitamin C as soon as they are peeled and cut.

Dilute orange juice for children—and for yourself if you're sensitive to sugar. Or fill an ice cube tray with orange juice to make orange ice cubes: Pop one into a glass of water for a subtle orange flavor and a shot of vitamin C with just a small amount of added natural sugar.

Makes about 16 ounces (470 milliliters)

5 medium oranges (about 2½ pounds/1.25 kilograms), cut in half

[139]

Press the orange halves through a citrus press. (Alternatively, you can peel the oranges and run them through a juicer.) Pour into glasses and serve, over ice if you like, or pour into a container, cover, and keep in the refrigerator until ready to use.

AROMATHERAPY IN ACTION

After you juice your oranges, passing the peels down the garbage disposal provides a perky citrus smell; no need to go out and buy orange essential oil to do the trick. The act of juicing oranges itself is instant aromatherapy: Some of the lively olfactory benefits of orange include elevating mood, reducing blood pressure, and providing a sense of calm.

Gracious Grapefruit Juice

In the pre–Organic Avenue days, when I was away from my kitchen I would buy my own grapefruits and bring them over to the local juice bar for juicing, as organic grapefruit juice was a rarity because of the high per-fruit cost. Now that you've set your kitchen up for at-home juicing, grapefruit juice is an affordable option, so there's no need to pass over this powerful member of the citrus family. You wouldn't want to miss out on its incredible nutrient profile: Grapefruit contains vitamins C, A, B-complex, and E, calcium, folic acid, potassium, and flavonoids and is known to be effective in the prevention of the common cold, diabetes, digestive disorders, fatigue, fever, and insomnia.

As with orange juice, dilute grapefruit juice for children—and for yourself if you're sensitive to sugar—or enjoy a whole grapefruit, pith and all, for a dose of regulating fiber. Note that grapefruit is contraindicated while taking certain prescriptions; check with your doctor if you are unsure.

Makes about 16 ounces (470 milliliters)

4 medium grapefruits (about 2½ pounds/1.25 kilograms), cut in half

[140]

Press the grapefruit halves through a citrus press. (Alternatively, you can peel the grapefruits and run them through a juicer.) Pour into glasses and serve, over ice if you like, or pour into a container, cover, and keep in the refrigerator until ready to use.

DID YOU KNOW?

Pink and red grapefruits are rich in the antioxidant lycopene, the same antioxidant found in tomatoes that's widely lauded for its anticancer properties, particularly against prostate cancer. (White grapefruit does not contain lycopene.) Other lycopene-containing fruits: apricots, watermelon, papaya, guava, and persimmon. Tropical fruit juice, anyone?

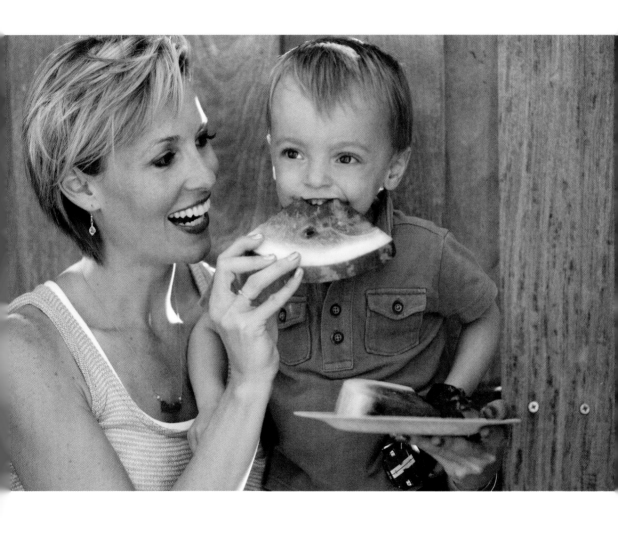

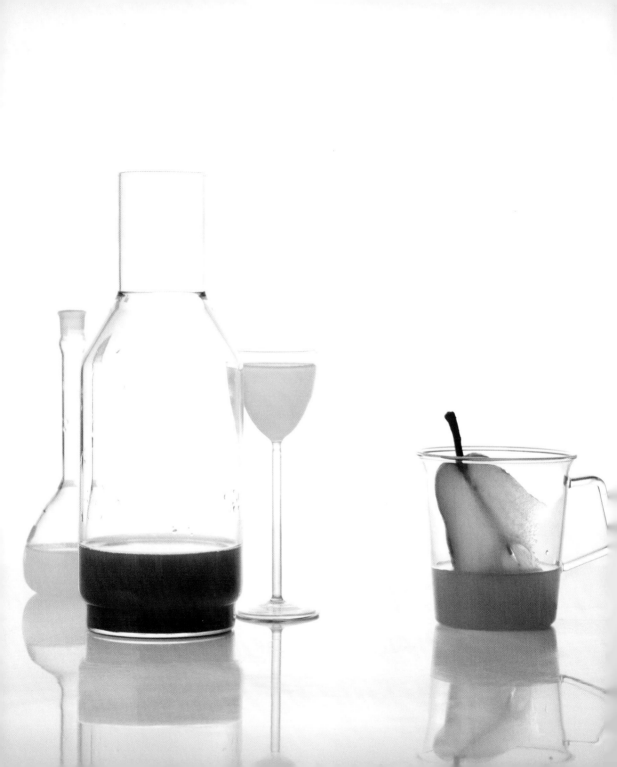

Precious Pear Juice

Pears tend to be neglected in the juicing world. We at Organic Avenue are working to change that by offering pear juice on our menu and showing you how to make your own at home. Once you taste fresh unpasteurized pear juice—rich, thick, and sweet—you won't believe what you've been missing. And you'll want to make some for your kids: Pears are often recommended for young children because of their hypoallergenic qualities.

Some more reasons to feel good about pear juice: The pectin in pears is a diuretic, and drinking pear juice has a mild laxative effect, keeping you regular. Pears are anti-inflammatory and high in antioxidants, making pear juice a good choice when you feel a cold coming on. Pears truly do pack a punch, as they also contain vitamins A, B_1, B_2, C, E, folic acid, and niacin as well as copper, phosphorus, and potassium.

Makes about 16 ounces (470 milliliters)

6 medium pears (about 2½ pounds/1.15 kilograms), stemmed and cut into
  quarters

[143]

Run the pears through a juicer. Pour into glasses and serve, over ice if you like, or pour into a container, cover, and keep in the refrigerator until ready to use.

A WORD ON ORGANIC JUICING

In the early days of transitioning to a LOVE*-based living foods diet, the importance of eating organic quickly became apparent to me. Especially in the juicing department: By liquefying your fruits and veggies, you are packing in the produce, a concentrated blast of nutrition; what you don't want is an additional blast of concentrated GMOs and pesticides. Again, you are doing good for yourself *and* the planet as you vote with your dollars for cleaner soil, food, and water, and ultimately a cleaner you.

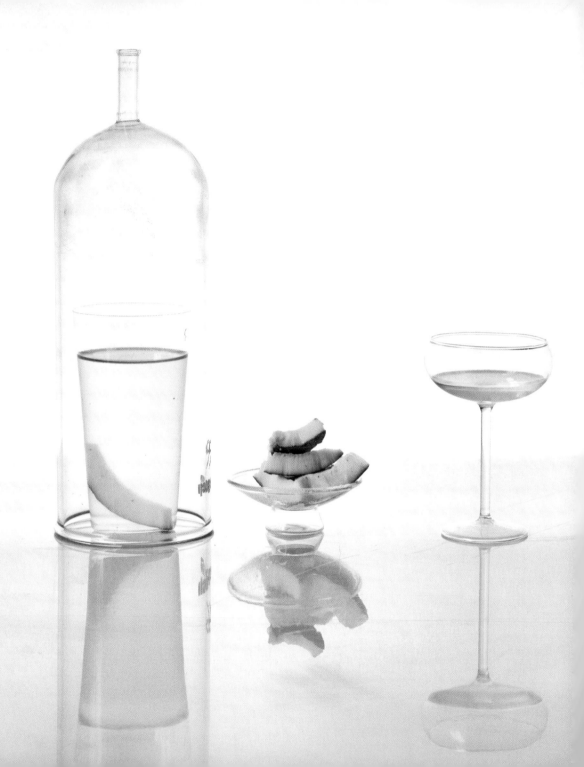

Clearly Coconut Water

My son, Oliver, simply calls it "juice." It's the beverage he regularly asks for, and I happily serve it to him, diluted with water for his young system. I think of all the nourishment he is getting: Coconut water has been credited with everything from fighting viruses to balancing pH, improving circulation, and boosting metabolism. And coconut water has amazing properties of hydration; in fact, the coconut palm tree works hard for that to happen: The tree filters the water through its roots in the soil from several feet away and pulls it through the trunk out into the branches over a several-month period and fills the seed with luscious clean water for us to enjoy. FYI: Coconut water is what you find when you break open the coconut; coconut *milk*, on the other hand, is made from the flesh of the coconut, blended to extract the liquid (see our Creamy Coconut Mylk recipe, page 189). For recipes that call for Clearly Coconut Water, bottled can be substituted as a time-saver—just make sure the bottle is labeled "raw" or "unpasteurized" and avoid anything found in a shelf-stable box.

Makes about 10 ounces (300 milliliters)

1 young coconut   [145]

Crack open the coconut and pour out the coconut water, as indicated on the following page, reserving the meat for another recipe or to eat out of hand.

HOW TO OPEN A YOUNG COCONUT

Young coconuts are the coconut of choice for those following the LOVE*Lifestyle, as they are higher in nutrition and full of healthy fats, and their soft flesh is extremely adaptable; we use it in blended drinks such as Creamy Coconut Mylk (page 189), to make yogurt and other desserts, and to enjoy scooped right out of the shell. A young coconut is off-white in color with a pointy top (as opposed to the more common-to-supermarkets mature coconut, which has a dark brown, hairy hard shell).

Here's how to open a young coconut and enjoy its flesh and water. The number one tip is to be super-cautious at all times and watch your fingers when you cut!

- Place the coconut on a sturdy, flat work surface.
- Hold one side of the coconut with one hand, and using a heavy knife or cleaver, make a horizontal cut on the opposite side of the coconut about one third into the coconut and about 1 inch below the tip, with the blade at a 45-degree angle. Your goal is to break into the inner shell.
- Give the coconut a quarter turn and make another cut like the first, connecting the second cut to the first (if it doesn't connect, give it another whack or two until it does).
- Continue twice more, giving the coconut two more quarter turns, cutting each time to connect with the previous cut, until you have cut a square off the tip. Using the bottom of the knife's blade, pry the top open.
- Pour the water into a pitcher, glass, or blender, depending on the recipe. (Or pull up a straw and drink right from the fruit, tropical style.)
- Turn the coconut on its side and break it open with the knife, holding the knife at a 45-degree angle and hitting it hard so the knife gets stuck in the coconut. Now slam the coconut on its side (with the knife still in the coconut) until it splits in half. Spoon out and enjoy the coconut meat or use it to make Creamy Coconut Mylk.

CLEARLY COCONUT ICE CUBES

Freeze coconut water in ice cube trays and toss a few into the fruit or vegetable juice of your choice for a hint of sweetness on-the-rocks style.

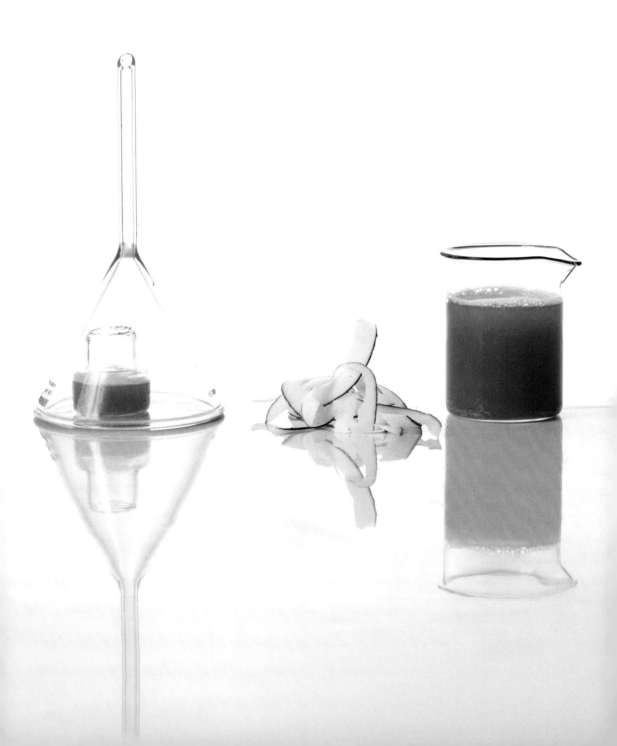

Crazy LOVE* Juice

You know how chocoholics like to say, "This would be even better if you added chocolate"? Well, at Organic Avenue our idea of upgrading any food or drink is to add something green. Here we did just that by combining greens with Clearly Coconut Water (page 145) to make Crazy LOVE*. We love the match it makes: The intensity of the chlorophyll-rich bitter greens plays off the sweetness of the coconut, pleasing your taste buds while oxygenating your blood and keeping your system hydrated. Great as a pre- or post-workout beverage.

Makes about 14 ounces (420 milliliters)

4 kale leaves, including stems
4 romaine lettuce leaves
Handful of spinach leaves
1 unpeeled cucumber, ends trimmed and roughly chopped
1 cup (240 milliliters) Clearly Coconut Water (page 145) or bottled raw coconut
  water

Run the kale, lettuce, spinach, and cucumber through a juicer, then add the coconut water. Pour into glasses and serve, over ice if you like, or pour into a container, cover, and keep in the refrigerator until ready to serve.

[149]

Variation: Crazy LOVE* with Lime
Run 1 peeled lime through the juicer with the rest of the ingredients.

GREEN IT UP
Just as we did here with our Crazy LOVE*, you can add a handful of greens to *any* non-green drink for a nice hit of chlorophyll.

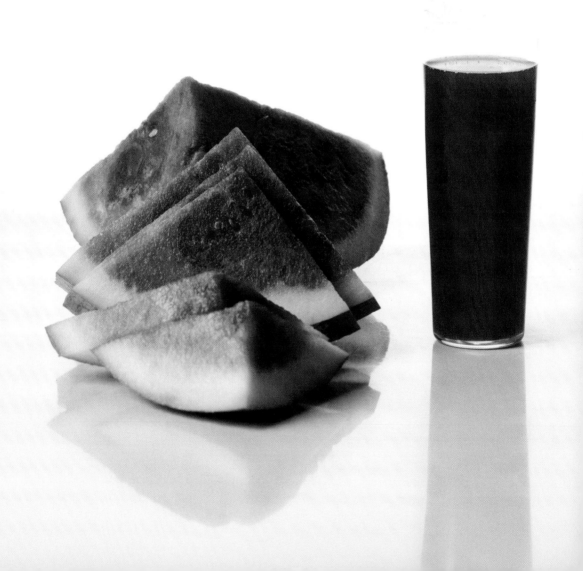

Wonderful Watermelon Juice

Watermelon, sweet treat that it is, is in fact more than 90 percent water, making watermelon juice a wonderfully hydrating low-sugar beverage, perfect for sipping generously poolside, keeping you cool and comfortable. Look for watermelons that are heavy for their size to ensure maximum juiciness.

Makes about 16 ounces (470 milliliters)

4 cups (650 grams) watermelon chunks

Run the watermelon through a juicer (you can run the rind through too, for a chlorophyll boost). Pour into glasses and serve, over ice if you like, or pour into a container, cover, and keep in the refrigerator until ready to use.

DID YOU KNOW?
Most juices marked "from concentrate" are reconstituted with water, at best filtered tap water from municipal water facilities in industrial zones. Another reason fresh is best.

[151]

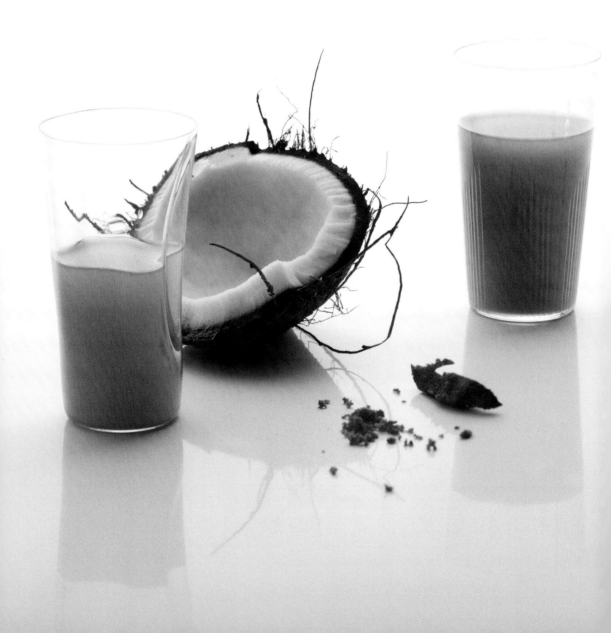

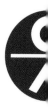

Tonics

Organic Avenue Tonics are elixirs, unique water-based drinks with powerful ingredients like turmeric, ginger, lemon, and cayenne added in large, medicinal amounts. Tonics are at once intensely flavored and light and refreshing; they'll make you pucker, they'll quench a post-workout thirst, they'll aim to heal what ails you. Grab one and prepare for a new experience!

[153]

Opposite: Truth Tonic (page 156)

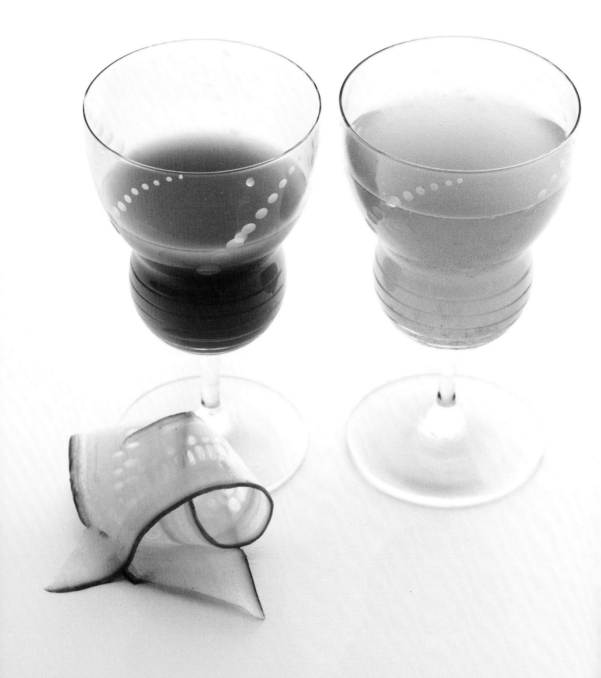

Generous Ginger Lemonade

This sweet-tart tonic, generous with the ginger, is intense yet refreshing, just the thing to keep your immune system mellow and content all year long. Slightly warmed, it's a flu-season tonic; ice cold, it quenches a deep summer thirst; keep a bottle by your side to counter motion sickness when you're on the road.

Most lemonade is filled with sugar and contains only traces of lemon; Organic Avenue's version contains a blend of lemon and lime with just enough natural coconut sugar to keep your lips from puckering. And the warmth of the ginger balances the brightness of the citrus, taking our lemonade to a whole new level.

Makes a little more than 16 ounces (470 milliliters)

2 cups (470 milliliters) water
½ lemon, peeled and seeded
½ lime, peeled and seeded
¼ cup (30 grams) coconut sugar
1-inch (1.25-centimeter) piece ginger

[155]

Combine all the ingredients in a blender and blend at high speed until smooth. Strain through a fine-mesh strainer, pressing on the solids to extract all the liquid, then pour into glasses and serve, over ice if you like, or pour into a container, cover, and keep in the refrigerator until ready to use.

Truth Tonic

Why make a tonic out of turmeric? The reasons are varied and quite convincing. Let's start with a big one: This orange-colored spice from the ginger family is liberally used in Indian cooking, where the rate of Alzheimer's is about 1 percent in people aged sixty-five and over (in the United States it's 13 percent). Researchers attribute this dramatically lower number in part to turmeric and its brain-supporting active ingredient, curcumin. In fact, turmeric has been used in Indian Ayurvedic medicine for centuries for fighting infections and supporting all body systems. We in the West are beginning to catch on. So, really, why *not* make a tonic out of turmeric?

Makes 16 ounces (470 milliliters)

2 cups (470 milliliters) water
½ lemon, peeled and seeded
1-inch (2.5-centimeter) piece fresh turmeric
¼ cup (30 grams) coconut sugar
Pinch of ground cayenne
Pinch of salt

Combine all the ingredients in a blender and blend at high speed until smooth. Strain through a fine-mesh strainer, pressing on the solids to extract all the liquid, then pour into glasses and serve, over ice if you like, or pour into a container, cover, and keep in the refrigerator until ready to use.

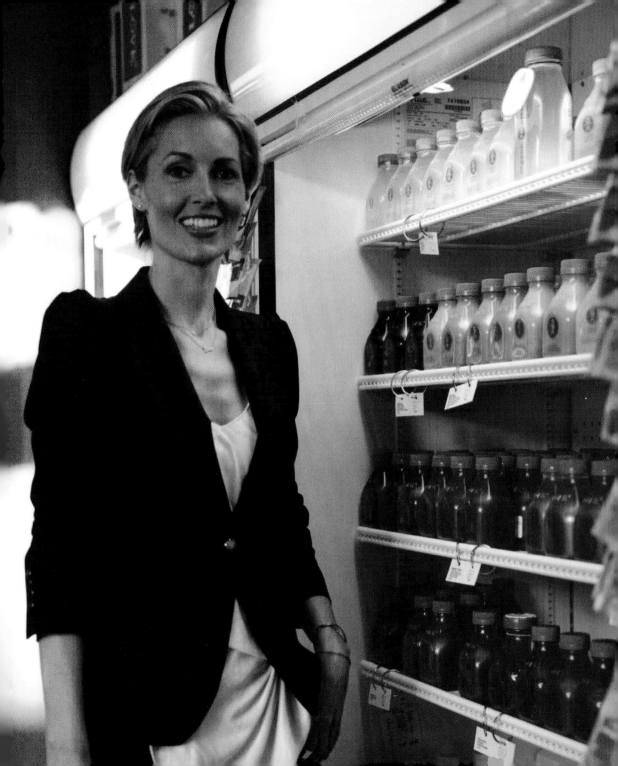

Master Tonic

Is super-cleansing your goal? Mission accomplished with this sweet, tart, and spicy mix of lemon, cayenne, and coconut sugar that will hydrate you while detoxing the whole system. Blending the whole peeled lemon, pith and all, makes for a tart treat; those with sweeter palates can add more coconut sugar or try substituting milder plain fresh-squeezed lemon juice for the blended lemon.

Makes a little more than 16 ounces (470 milliliters)

2 cups (470 milliliters) water
1 lemon, peeled and seeded
¼ cup (30 grams) coconut sugar, or more as needed
Pinch of ground cayenne

Combine all the ingredients in a blender and blend at high speed until smooth. Strain through a fine-mesh strainer, pressing on the solids to extract all the liquid, then pour into glasses and serve, over ice if you like, or pour into a container, cover, and keep in the refrigerator until ready to use.

❜❜ *Don't give up on LOVE*. You may at some point be tempted to reexperience the pleasure and pain of the other side, yet once you get good and familiar with the health, youth, energy, and vitality you can experience on a committed LOVE*Lifestyle, you will know where home is and always head back."*

—DENISE MARI

Grateful Green Lemonade

Here we've turned our Generous Ginger Lemonade (page 155) green by adding spinach and cucumber. Another way to broaden your juicing options and help the world go a little more green!

Makes a little more than 16 ounces (470 milliliters)

Generous Ginger Lemonade (page 155)
½ cucumber, end trimmed and roughly chopped
Handful of spinach leaves

Combine all the ingredients in a blender and blend at high speed until smooth. Strain through a fine-mesh strainer, pressing on the solids to extract all the liquid, then pour into glasses and serve, over ice if you like, or pour into a container, cover, and keep in the refrigerator until ready to use.

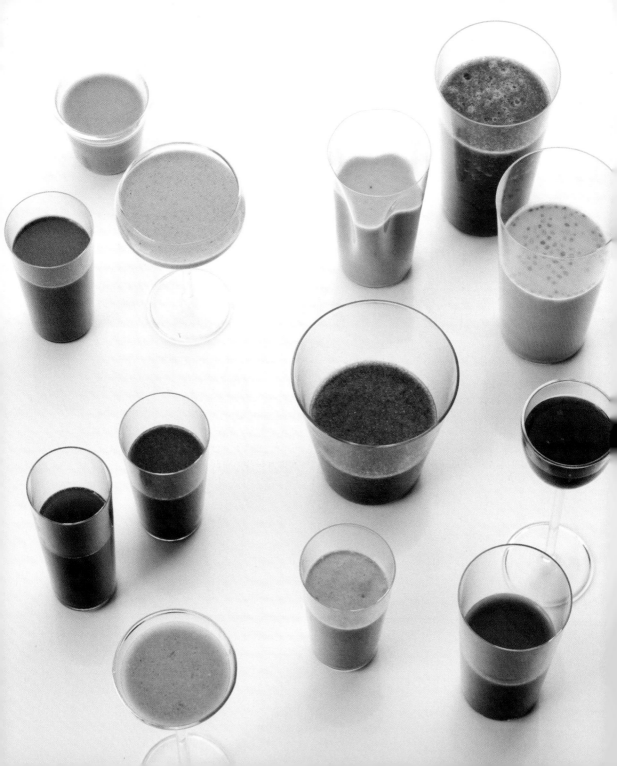

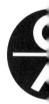

Smoothies

Smoothies are a meal in a glass, with whole fruits, veggies, nuts, and other ingredients blended with the fiber intact, keeping you full and satiated till you next sit down to eat (or drink, if you're staying liquid). Follow the Organic Avenue smoothie recipes as directed, or use them as starting points for smoothies of your own creation. Some ideas to get you going:

- Increase the greens for a more savory experience.
- Subtract the chocolate when you're deeply cleansing.
- Use what you have on hand and what you LOVE*, with a coconut water or mylk (page 145 or 189) base and banana and/or dates and coconut sugar for sweetness as a good place to start.
- If you like your smoothies super-smooth, strain them before serving.
- If you like your smoothies super-frothy, use frozen fruit as your base or freeze coconut water in ice cube trays and blend them into your drink in place of liquid coconut water.
- Add water, coconut water, or nut mylk of your choice to thin overly thick smoothies.

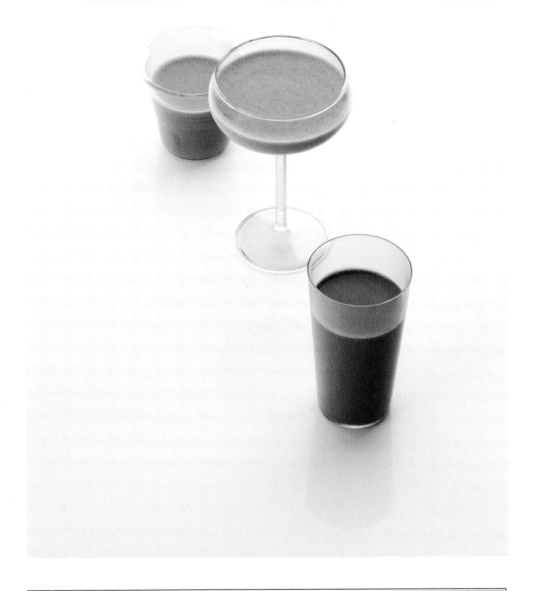

NOTE

We use vanilla powder rather than vanilla extract because vanilla powder is alcohol-free and available in its raw state; you can find it in some natural food stores and online.

Cheerful Chai Smoothie

Here we start with a base of Creative Cashew Mylk and add warming spices to offer you a noncaffeinated version of the traditional tea-based drink. You won't need the caffeine, because according to Indian Ayurvedic medicine, chai spices are considered both calming and mentally invigorating as well as overall health enhancers: cardamom is known to be a mood elevator; cinnamon counters fatigue; nutmeg, ginger, and cloves help with digestion; and black pepper has antioxidant properties. The spice blend recipe makes enough for multiple smoothies; keep a jar of it near your blender for whenever you get the urge.

Makes about 16 ounces (470 milliliters)

2 cups (470 milliliters) Creative Cashew Mylk (page 187)
2 dates, soaked in water to cover for 2 to 3 hours, drained, and pitted
2 teaspoons lucuma powder
¾ teaspoon Chai Spice Blend (recipe follows)
¼ teaspoon vanilla powder (see Note)

Combine all the ingredients in a blender and blend at high speed until smooth. [163]
Pour into glasses and serve, over ice if you like, or pour into a container, cover, and keep in the refrigerator until ready to use.

Chai Spice Blend
Makes just under ¼ cup (20 grams)

2 tablespoons ground cardamom
1 tablespoon ground cinnamon
¾ teaspoon freshly grated nutmeg
¾ teaspoon ground ginger
⅛ teaspoon ground cloves
⅛ teaspoon freshly ground black pepper

Combine all the ingredients in a small bowl; store in a spice jar.

Cherished Chocolate Smoothie

Dessert in a glass: This smoothie is rich and decadent-tasting, with all the wonderful antioxidant, anti-aging properties of raw chocolate, plus omega-3-rich hemp seeds and protein-packed cashews. So get your chocolate fix here, all the while packing your body with a potent free radical–fighting punch!

Makes 16 ounces (470 milliliters)

2 cups (470 milliliters) Creative Cashew Mylk (page 187)
4 dates, soaked in water to cover for 2 to 3 hours, drained, and pitted
¼ cup (18 grams) cocoa powder
½ teaspoon vanilla powder (see Note, page 162)

Combine all the ingredients in a blender and blend at high speed until smooth. Pour into glasses and serve, over ice if you like, or pour into a container, cover, and keep in the refrigerator until ready to use.

Champion Chocolate Smoothie

Like a liquefied nutty candy bar, but good for you, with a triple shot of protein and just the right amount of chocolate to bring a smile to your face.

Makes about 16 ounces (470 milliliters)

1½ cups (350 milliliters) Appealing Almond Mylk (page 185)
1 large ripe fresh or frozen banana, broken into pieces
4 to 5 dates, soaked in water to cover for 2 to 3 hours, drained, and pitted
3 tablespoons coconut sugar
2 tablespoons almond butter
2 tablespoons vegan protein powder, such as Boku brand
2 tablespoons cocoa powder
1 tablespoon coconut oil
1 tablespoon cacao nibs
¼ teaspoon vanilla powder (see Note, page 162)
Pinch of salt

Combine all the ingredients in a blender and blend at high speed until smooth. Pour into glasses and serve, over ice if you like, or pour into a container, cover, and keep in the refrigerator until ready to use.

[165]

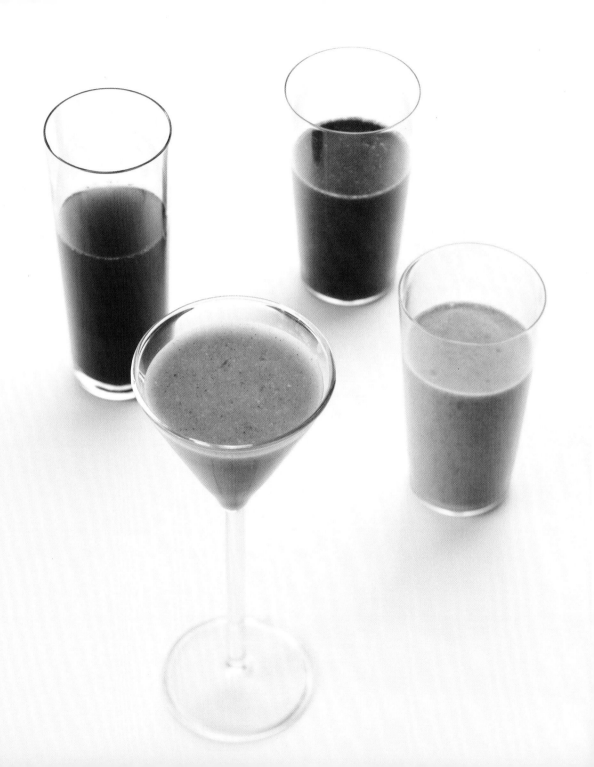

Courageous Chocolate Mint Smoothie

This smoothie features crunchy cacao nibs and is topped off with a few drops of peppermint oil for a cooling sensation and a digestive boost. The mint, along with the raw cacao, hemp seeds, and cashews, provides satisfying yet refreshing relief during the sultry days of summer.

Makes about 16 ounces (470 milliliters)

2 cups (470 milliliters) Creative Cashew Mylk (page 187)
4 dates, soaked in water to cover for 2 to 3 hours, drained, and pitted
¼ cup (25 grams) cacao nibs
½ teaspoon peppermint extract

Combine all the ingredients in a blender and blend at high speed until smooth. Pour into glasses and serve, over ice if you like, or pour into a container, cover, and keep in the refrigerator until ready to use.

[167]

DID YOU KNOW?

Mint oil (in peppermint extract) is known for its nerve-calming and mind-opening properties, giving you at once a boost of alertness and a feeling of calmness. It also is known to relieve headaches.

Outrageously Orange Smoothie

Reminiscent of the childhood favorite frozen orange treat on a stick, but with the fresh, clean flavor of 100 percent real orange and dairy-free coconut meat serving as your nondairy cream. If you're not already pulling out the juicer as a daily ritual, feel free to use prepared freshly pressed orange juice as a time-saver. And if this one becomes a regular in your smoothie rotation, you'll save even more time by employing this tip: Keep individual serving packets of the dry ingredients in small containers or plastic bags, label them, and when you're ready to make your smoothie, just empty one into a blender, add the OJ and coconut, and you're ready to blend.

Makes about 16 ounces (470 milliliters)

3 oranges, peeled and segmented, or 1 cup (240 milliliters) fresh orange juice
⅓ cup (60 grams) packed fresh coconut meat (see page 146)
2 tablespoons lucuma powder
2 tablespoons coconut sugar
¼ teaspoon vanilla powder (see Note, page 162)
Pinch of ground turmeric
Pinch of salt
Pinch of stevia powder

[168]

If you are starting with orange segments, run the oranges through a juicer, then combine all the ingredients in a blender and blend at high speed until smooth. Pour into glasses and serve, over ice if you like, or pour into a container, cover, and keep in the refrigerator until ready to serve.

DID YOU KNOW?

Oranges have more than 170 phytonutrients and are rich in flavonoids. One such flavonoid, hesperidin, stands out in its ability to augment the effect of vitamin C in the body (of which you'll be getting plenty in your OJ); it also has been shown to regulate cholesterol and blood pressure and provide significant antioxidant benefits. Oranges also have anticancer properties, particularly in relation to colon, stomach, and esophageal cancer. Now that's what I call sweet medicine!

Chocolate Banana Orange Protein Smoothie

Starting out with one of the best-ever smoothie combinations—banana and chocolate—this one gets even better with a splash of orange juice, finishing it off on a citrus high note. Cacao nibs add a fun crunch.

Makes about 16 ounces (470 milliliters)

½ orange, peeled and segmented, or 2 tablespoons fresh orange juice
¾ cup (175 milliliters) Clearly Coconut Water (page 145) or bottled raw
  coconut water
1 ripe frozen or fresh banana, broken into chunks
2 to 3 dates, soaked in water to cover for 2 to 3 hours, drained, and pitted
2 tablespoons vegan protein powder, such as Boku brand
3 tablespoons cocoa powder
2 tablespoons coconut sugar
1 tablespoon cacao nibs
1 teaspoon coconut oil
⅛ teaspoon ground cinnamon
Pinch of salt

If you're starting with orange segments, run them through a juicer, then combine all the ingredients in a blender and blend at high speed until smooth. Pour into glasses and serve, over ice if you like, or pour into a container, cover, and keep in the refrigerator until ready to serve.

Glorious Green Blueberry Protein Smoothie

When you're looking for a smoothie that's full of protein but also want to get your daily greens in, this one, with its trio of protein sources and generous amounts of greens, is for you. Berries and dates sweeten the deal, and lemon juice adds a note of lightness.

Makes about 16 ounces (470 milliliters)

1 cup (240 milliliters) Clearly Coconut Water (page 145) or bottled raw coconut water
½ cup (50 grams) fresh or frozen blueberries
½ medium unpeeled cucumber, end trimmed and roughly chopped
1 large collard green leaf, including stem, torn into pieces
1 large kale leaf, including stem, torn into pieces
2 mint leaves
2 dates, soaked in water to cover for 2 to 3 hours, drained, and pitted
1 tablespoon fresh lemon juice
2 tablespoons vegan protein powder, such as Boku brand
2 tablespoons coconut sugar
1 tablespoon supergreen powder, such as Boku brand
¼ teaspoon spirulina powder
Pinch of salt

[171]

Combine all the ingredients in a blender and blend at high speed until smooth. Pour into glasses and serve, over ice if you like, or pour into a container, cover, and keep in the refrigerator until ready to serve.

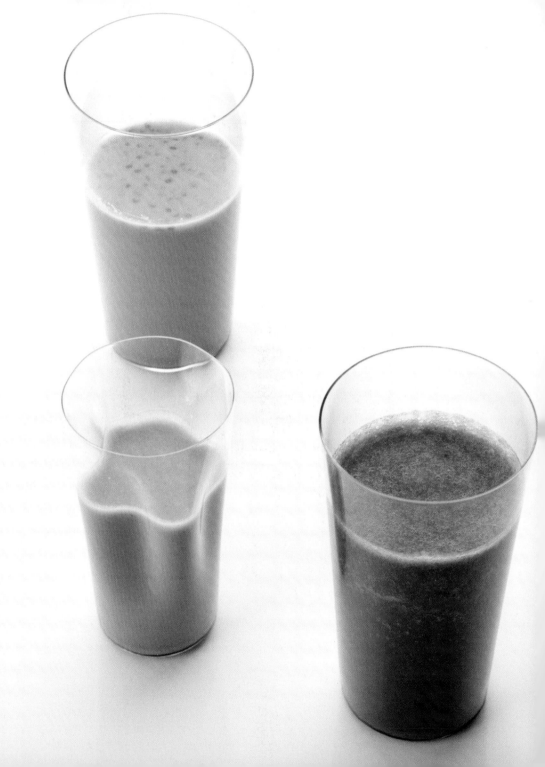

Lively Lemon-Lime Smoothie

Get ready to pucker! Juicing the lemon and lime, peel and all, provides added bioflavonoid benefits, including anti-inflammatory and antioxidant effects, and gives a pumped-up citrus experience. To save time and for a slightly mellower experience, hand-squeeze your lemon and lime rather than running them through the juicer. Super-sweet stevia offsets the sourness without adding calories or affecting your blood sugar. Freeze the coconut meat for a frostier shake.

Makes about 16 ounces (470 milliliters)

½ unpeeled lime or juice of 1 lime
½ unpeeled lemon or juice of 1 lemon
1½ cups (350 milliliters) water
½ avocado, peeled and pitted
¼ medium unpeeled cucumber (50 grams), end trimmed and roughly chopped
½ cup (70 grams) packed fresh coconut meat (see page 146)
½ teaspoon stevia powder
Pinch of salt

[173]

If you are starting with lime and lemon halves, run them through a juicer, then combine all the ingredients in a blender and blend at high speed until smooth. Pour into glasses and serve, over ice if you like, or pour into a container, cover, and keep in the refrigerator until you are ready to serve.

ACID TASTE, ALKALINE EFFECT
Although lemon and lime have an acidic taste, they actually have an alkaline reaction upon digestion; in fact, they can have a profound effect on the treatment of acidity in the digestive system. The same is true for grapefruit. See page 11 for more on the importance of an alkaline body.

Magical Matcha Chia Smoothie

Matcha is no ordinary green tea: When you drink matcha, you are drinking the whole leaf, not just the brewed water, giving you about ten times the antioxidant power of other green teas. Matcha is also high in vitamins and other nutrients and is a powerful cancer fighter and fat burner. It is also said to have an anti-aging effect: In Okinawa, Japan, where some of the longest-living population resides, matcha tea is a staple. It is available in tea shops, Japanese groceries, and some natural food stores.

And chia seeds, full of fiber and omega-3 fatty acids, are magicians of hydration, able to absorb more than twelve times their weight in liquid, which is why we love them so much at Organic Avenue. They give your body the prolonged power you need while you're working out or clearing out with one of the LOVE*Cleanses. Coconut blossom sugar is a lighter, creamy form of coconut sugar that keeps the color of the drink bright (see Food and Equipment Sources, page 317). If it's not available, granulated coconut sugar will work fine.

Makes about 16 ounces (470 milliliters)

[174]

1¾ cups (420 milliliters) water
¼ cup (35 grams) pumpkin seeds
2½ teaspoons matcha tea powder
¼ cup (115 grams) coconut blossom sugar
1½ teaspoons Cleansing Chlorophyll Booster Shot (page 111)
½ teaspoon vanilla powder (see Note, page 162)
Pinch of ground cardamom
Pinch of ground cinnamon
Pinch of salt
1½ tablespoons chia seeds

Combine all the ingredients except the chia seeds in a blender and blend on high speed until smooth. Transfer to a pitcher, whisk in the chia seeds, and let the mixture sit in the refrigerator, stirring occasionally, until the chia seeds swell, about 2 hours. Pour into glasses and serve, over ice if you like, or pour into a container, cover, and keep in the refrigerator until ready to use.

CALM AND CLEAR WITH MATCHA

Yes, matcha contains caffeine, but it also contains L-theanine, an amino acid that promotes relaxation, so it won't give you that jittery high followed by the inevitable crash many of us experience after the afternoon coffee break. Take it from the Japanese Zen Buddhist monks, who traditionally have drunk it to remain alert but calm during their long hours spent in meditation.

Green Gone Bananas Smoothie

Greens and bananas: sweet yet savory, creamy yet earthy, and a great way to get the greens in. Freeze overripe bananas in bulk for multiple batches.

Makes about 14 ounces (420 milliliters)

1½ cups (350 milliliters) Clearly Coconut Water (page 145) or bottled raw
   coconut water
1 large kale leaf, including stem, torn into pieces
2 medium ripe fresh or frozen bananas, broken into pieces
2 tablespoons coconut sugar
¼ teaspoon spirulina powder

Combine all the ingredients in a blender and blend at high speed until smooth. Pour into glasses and serve, over ice if you like, or pour into a container, cover, and keep in the refrigerator until ready to use.

[176]

Green Embrace Smoothie

Mango adds its characteristic sweetness to counter the deep, dark greenness of this superfood-heavy shake. Substitute coconut water for the plain water for extra sweetness and bonus electrolytes.

Makes about 16 ounces (470 milliliters)

1 cup (240 milliliters) water
1 ripe frozen or fresh banana, broken into chunks
Handful of spinach leaves
½ medium mango, peeled, pitted, and roughly chopped
2 teaspoons coconut oil
1 teaspoon supergreen powder, such as Boku brand
1 teaspoon lucuma powder
¼ teaspoon spirulina powder

Combine all the ingredients in a blender and blend at high speed until smooth. Pour into glasses and serve, over ice if you like, or pour into a container, cover, and keep in the refrigerator until ready to serve.

[177]

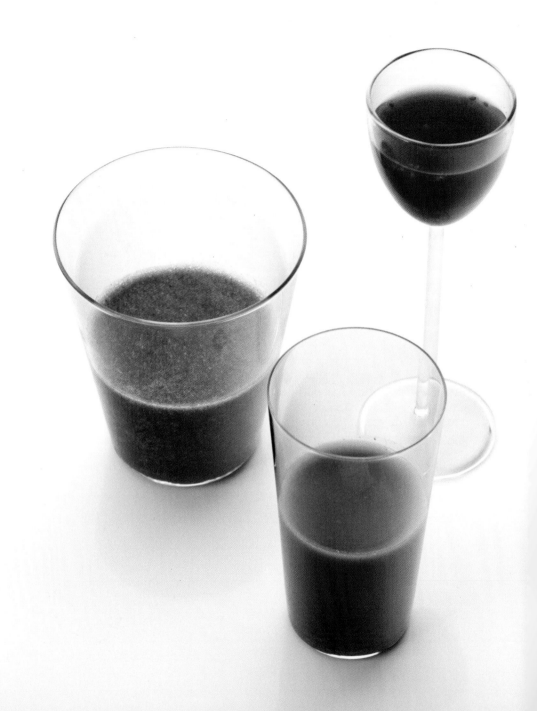

Blissful Berry Protein Smoothie

This purple-hued potion is as beautiful to look at as it is a delight to the taste buds, and it's also an excellent protein supplement. You really can't go wrong combining berries and bananas, and when you freeze them first, your reward is a frosty and extra-creamy smoothie. The base is mildly sweet coconut water, a natural for this tropical treat, but if you don't have coconut water handy, pure plain water will work just fine, as will any seasonal berry, such as raspberries or blackberries or a single berry. What you don't want to do without is the lemon juice: The splash of citrus helps bring out the flavor of the berries to the max.

Makes about 16 ounces (470 milliliters)

½ cup (120 milliliters) Clearly Coconut Water (page 145) or bottled raw
    coconut water
¼ cup (60 milliliters) water
1 ripe fresh or frozen banana, broken into chunks
1 cup (100 grams) fresh or frozen blueberries
¾ cup (100 grams) hulled fresh or frozen strawberries
2 dates, soaked in water to cover for 2 to 3 hours, drained, and pitted   [179]
2 tablespoons vegan protein powder, such as Boku brand
1 tablespoon fresh lemon juice
½ teaspoon coconut oil
¼ teaspoon vanilla powder (see Note, page 162)
Pinch of salt

Combine all the ingredients in a blender and blend at high speed until smooth. Pour into glasses and serve, over ice if you like, or pour into a container, cover, and keep in the refrigerator until ready to serve.

Healthy Hibiscus Chia Smoothie

Hydrating, omega-3-rich chia seeds make another appearance here, added to wine-red-colored antioxidant-rich hibiscus tea, made from the sweet-tart hibiscus flower, common to Mexico, Latin America, and North Africa. You can find the powder in herb stores or Latino grocery stores; if only the dried whole flowers are available, grind them in a blender or spice grinder to pulverize them. In a pinch, simply rip open a hibiscus tea bag and go from there.

Makes about 20 ounces (600 milliliters)

2½ cups (600 milliliters) water
½ cup (60 grams) coconut sugar
1½ tablespoons fresh lemon juice
1½ teaspoons hibiscus powder
4 mint leaves, torn
3 tablespoons chia seeds

In a blender, combine all the ingredients except the chia seeds and blend until smooth. Transfer to a pitcher, whisk in the chia seeds, and let the mixture sit in the refrigerator, stirring occasionally, until the chia seeds swell, about 2 hours. Pour into glasses and serve, over ice if you like, or pour into a container, cover, and keep in the refrigerator until ready to use.

UPPING YOUR HYDRATION WITH CHIA SEEDS

You can add chia seeds to any juice or smoothie for that extra hit of hydration and a boost of fiber as well. Just follow the instructions above, adding about 1 tablespoon chia seeds for every 1 cup (240 milliliters) liquid and letting your drink sit, stirring occasionally, for about 2 hours, until the chia seeds swell.

Blueberry Banana Spirulina Smoothie

Spirulina powder, a blue-green algae, is one of the richest, most concentrated sources of protein in the plant kingdom, and a complete protein to boot. It is an excellent energy source, high in beta-carotene and thus strengthening to the immune system, and full of B vitamins, iron, calcium, magnesium, and other trace minerals. Our advice for supplementing with spirulina: Combine it with something sweet, like the bananas and berries here, to counter its mossy, marinelike flavor (but rest assured there is literally nothing fishy about spirulina—it is 100 percent vegan).

Makes about 16 ounces (470 milliliters)

1 cup (240 milliliters) Clearly Coconut Water (page 145) or bottled raw coconut
   water
2 ripe fresh or frozen bananas, broken into chunks
1 cup (100 grams) fresh or frozen blueberries
2 tablespoons coconut oil
¼ teaspoon spirulina powder

[181]

Combine all the ingredients in a blender and blend at high speed until smooth. Pour into glasses and serve, over ice if you like, or pour into a container, cover, and keep in the refrigerator until ready to serve.

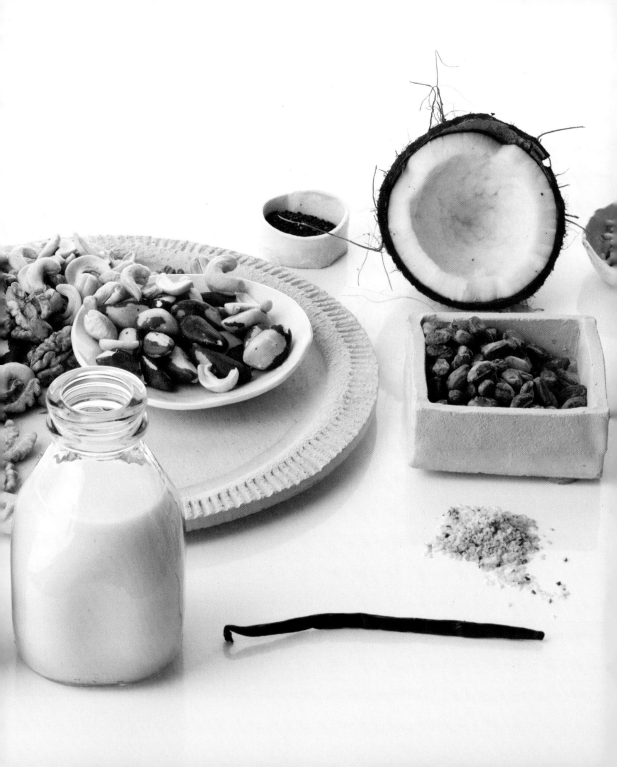

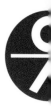

Mylks

Mylks are blended drinks, just like smoothies but based on nuts or coconut. Knock back a glass as is, with or without a vegan cookie for dunking, pour some over Gracious Granola (page 285), or use as the basis of a libation of your own creation.

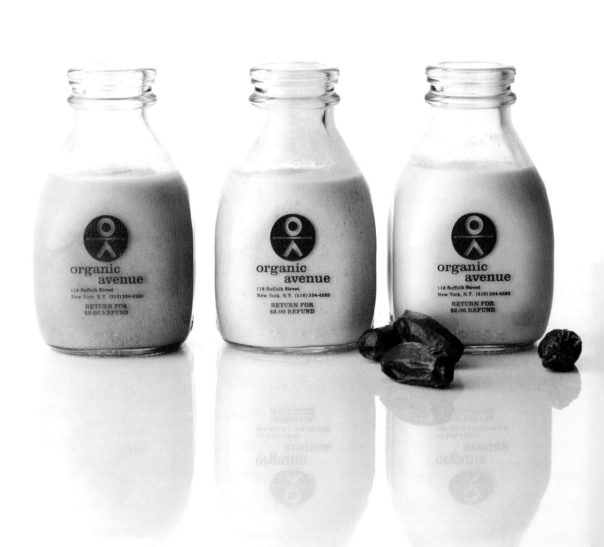

Appealing Almond Mylk

Almond Mylk, made by simply blending almonds with water and straining, is a protein-rich, slightly sweet superdrink, a superstar in the world of milk alternatives, with a glass of it containing significant B vitamins, iron, magnesium, zinc, and vitamin E. Best of all, Almond Mylk contains roughly the same amount of calcium as dairy milk, but with no mucous-forming lactose and just a fraction of the calories. So let's give a dairy-free round of applause for the little nut!

Makes about 1 quart (1 liter)

1⅔ cups (115 grams) raw almonds
4 cups (1 liter) water

In a medium bowl or right in your blender, soak the almonds overnight in water to cover. Drain and rinse the almonds, place them in the blender, and add the water. Blend at high speed until smooth, then strain through a nut milk bag or strainer lined with cheesecloth. Pour into glasses and serve, over ice if you like, or pour into a container, cover, and keep in the refrigerator until ready to use.

[185]

Variation: Valiant Vanilla Mylk

Add ½ teaspoon vanilla powder (see Note, page 162) to your Almond Mylk.

DID YOU KNOW?

Most boxed almond milks are pasteurized and contain significant added sugars. Why add all that sugar when almonds are naturally sweet? When you make your own Almond Mylk, you get to experience the true taste of the nut: pleasingly sweet, refreshing, with a light almond flavor. And in contrast to the sterile, pasteurized almond milk you find in a box (did you know that the dictionary definition of *pasteurization* includes the words "partial sterilization"?), when you make your Almond Mylk with "living," unpasteurized almonds, it will be, well, the opposite: totally raw and full of life!

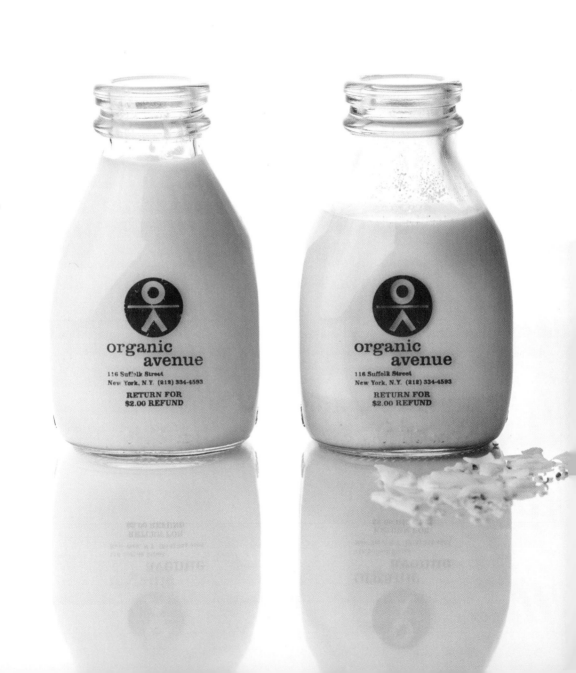

Creative Cashew Mylk

This is a foundation Organic Avenue recipe and the base for a trio of Organic Avenue favorites: Cheerful Chai Smoothie, Cherished Chocolate Smoothie, and Courageous Chocolate Mint Smoothie (pages 163, 164, and 167).

To save on cleanup, soak your cashews right in the blender, and to save on time, soak your nuts in advance or skip the soaking altogether—cashews are fairly soft and can be milked from their dry state; just make sure to turn your blender to its highest speed for the smoothest results. Extreme time-saver: Omit the Irish Moss Gel; your mylk will be a little thinner but equally delicious.

Makes about 1 quart (1 liter)

3½ cups (830 milliliters) water
⅓ cup (45 grams) cashews, soaked in water to cover overnight and drained
2 tablespoons hemp seeds
10 dates, soaked in water to cover for 2 to 3 hours, drained, and pitted
¼ cup Irish Moss Gel (optional; recipe follows)
Pinch of salt

[187]

Combine all the ingredients in a blender and blend at high speed until smooth. Pour into glasses and serve, over ice if you like, or pour into a container, cover, and keep in the refrigerator until ready to use.

Irish Moss Gel

Irish moss, also known as carrageen moss, is a seaweed with amazing thickening powers: Just soak and blend and this super algae transforms into a gel that gives body to your mylks and smoothies; it can also be used to emulsify salad dressings, thicken sauces, and lend desserts a creamy, light texture without added calories. You'll have leftover gel (you need to make the whole batch in order to get the blender to work its way through the dense moss), which will last for up to a week in the refrigerator or can be frozen for several months: Try popping premeasured portions into silicone muffin pans or ice cube trays so you will have them at the ready.

And Irish moss is not just filler; it's good for you too: It's used to ease respiratory issues, as it's soothing to the mucous membranes; it's full of antioxidants; it has high levels of iodine and other minerals; and it can even be used to soothe a sunburn or replenish wintry dry skin and chapped lips. To find it, see Food and Equipment Sources, page 317.

Makes about 1 quart (1 liter)

1 cup (120 grams) Irish moss
2 cups (470 milliliters) water

Place the Irish moss in a large bowl, add water to cover, and swirl it around a little to loosen any grit or sand from the moss. Drain, add fresh water to cover, cover with a dish towel, and soak overnight on the counter or up to 24 hours in the refrigerator. Drain and rinse very well to remove any remaining grit or sand. Place in a high-speed blender and add the 2 cups (470 milliliters) water. Blend on high speed until it turns into a smooth, gelatinous paste, stopping to pause a few times so your machine doesn't get overheated and scraping the sides of the machine a few times as necessary; add more water a little at a time if needed. Transfer to a container and store, covered, in the refrigerator.

Creamy Coconut Mylk

This recipe couldn't be easier—once you learn how to crack open a young coconut, which is pretty simple after you've practiced on a few. Then it's just a
matter of pouring out the coconut water, scooping out the flesh, and blending it
up. Young coconut, particularly young coconut water, has a long tradition in Indian healing systems; it's known for maintaining electrolyte balance (the water
has more electrolytes than any other natural food), preventing dehydration, and
purifying the blood. It's a rich treat—serve in tiny cups (try it in shot glasses!),
or drink a cup for breakfast and it will keep you on an energetic, no-slump high
all morning. Freeze the coconut flesh for a creamy mylk shake consistency.

Makes about 16 ounces (470 milliliters)

1 fresh young coconut

Crack open the coconut (see page 146). Drain the coconut water into a blender
and scoop the flesh of the coconut from the shell into the blender. Blend on
high speed until smooth. Pour into glasses and serve, over ice if you like, or
pour into a container, cover, and keep in the refrigerator until ready to use.

[189]

Sweet Strawberry Banana Mylk

This nostalgic, smile-inducing drink, flavored with strawberries plus a notice-able hint of lemon, is a favorite with kids, and adults love it for its honest taste, in another league from the artificially flavored stuff many of us grew up with. It's very important to use organic strawberries here (buy frozen if they are out of season), as conventional strawberries are heavily sprayed, so much so that they appear on the Environmental Working Group's "Dirty Dozen" list, our twelve most heavily sprayed fruits and vegetables (see ewg.org for the complete list).

Makes about 16 ounces (470 milliliters)

1 ripe banana, broken into chunks
1 cup (100 grams) frozen hulled strawberries
¾ cup (175 milliliters) Clearly Coconut Water (page 145) or bottled raw
    coconut water
½ cup (120 milliliters) Creative Cashew Mylk (page 187)
2 tablespoons fresh lemon juice
2 dates, soaked in water to cover for 2 to 3 hours, drained, and pitted
1 tablespoon coconut sugar (optional)
¼ teaspoon vanilla powder (see Note, page 162)
Pinch of salt

Combine all the ingredients in a blender and blend at high speed until smooth. Pour into glasses and serve, or pour into a container, cover, and keep in the refrigerator until ready to serve.

Grand Green Mylk

Here we turn Almond Mylk green by combining it with Mighty LOVE* Green Juice to ease you into the greens and to give those greens some extra protein—and you extra staying power as you go about your LOVE*-filled day.

Makes about 16 ounces (470 milliliters)

1 cup (240 milliliters) Mighty LOVE* Green Juice (page 127)
1 cup (240 milliliters) Appealing Almond Mylk (page 185)
¼ teaspoon ground cinnamon

Combine the Mighty LOVE* Green Juice and Almond Mylk in a pitcher and whisk in the cinnamon. Pour into glasses and serve, over ice if you like, or pour into a container, cover, and keep in the refrigerator until ready to use.

[191]

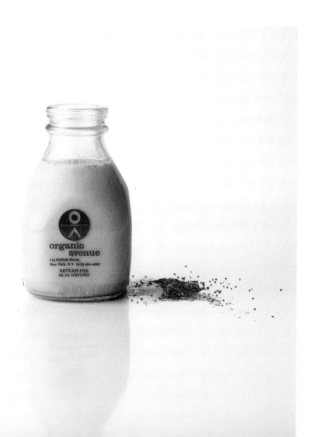

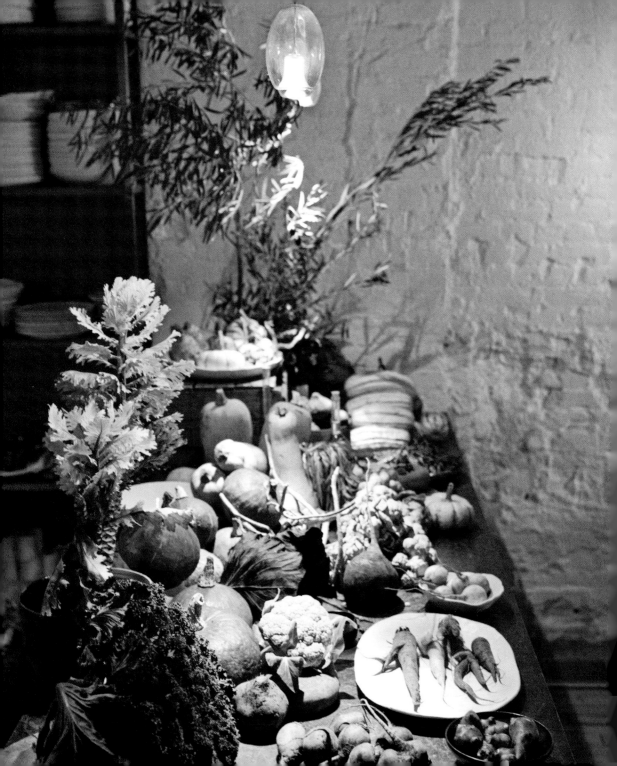

PART IV

The Food of LOVE*

Eating and cleansing go hand in hand in the world of LOVE*. Yes, you can go on Organic Avenue's juice-only LOVE*Cleanses (LOVE*Deep), but you can also choose a live food–containing cleanse (LOVE*Easy or LOVE*Fast), making our cleanses eminently compatible with everyday life. And here we'll give you backbone recipes to continue along your Live. Organic. Vegan. Experience. Everything from soup to nuts (salty, sweet, and crisped up in the dehydrator), with low-carb, gluten-free, live vegetable-based wraps and pasta dishes, even raw lasagna, salads both simple and sublime, nut-based cheeses, and puddings, cookies, and other delectable desserts. This is the moment we've all been waiting for. Let's eat!

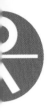

Salads and Dressings

At Organic Avenue, cleansing doesn't stop at the juicer; indulging in daily salads with all their health-promoting fiber is one of the best ways of continuing with your cleanse. In fact, salads are an integral part of the cleansing program itself (see the cleanse menus on pages 67 to 69).

Organic Avenue salads are not just tasty, they are downright *exciting*. Using exotic ingredients such as preserved lemons; flavor-enhancing components such as olives, capers, and raisins; and cheeses made from cashews and macadamias, they go far beyond the standard bowl of greens. And, in our experience, what separates a good salad from a great salad is the dressing, so we've pulled out the stops, with recipes including a simple but flavor-packed herb vinaigrette, a rich and creamy ranch dressing, and a more involved tzatziki dressing made from homemade cashew yogurt, to name a few.

Feel free to mix and match the dressings and salads according to what you have in the house or what's in season or available at the market. You can simplify a recipe by omitting labor-intensive ingredients such as the made-from-scratch cheeses, and if you're really short on time, you won't go wrong with a two-minute dressing boldly flavored with lemon juice or raw cider vinegar, good olive oil, and salt and pepper (note: skimping on the seasonings, especially salt, makes for a humdrum salad). Taste your dressing on a lettuce leaf or other salad ingredient before tossing—doing so will tell you not just how the dressing tastes, but how it will taste on the salad—and adjust the seasonings as needed.

When it comes to shopping for your salad ingredients, the great thing is that you can get many of them just about anywhere, be it your farmers' market, natural food store, or local supermarket (many have organic options nowadays), making salad a can-do-for-dinner option that most people can pull off any day of the week.

Big Greek Salad with Tzatziki Dressing

When you're looking for a salad as a meal, Greek salad—with its hearty vegetables, olives, and signature feta cheese topping—is an excellent choice. This is a unique Greek salad, because the feta cheese—made from macadamias and cashews—is completely vegan. And the tzatziki dressing, based on the yogurt and cucumber Greek appetizer of the same name, is also a vegan version, made with cashew yogurt in place of dairy yogurt. While this is one of the more involved salads in the Organic Avenue repertoire, you can easily simplify it by substituting the Lemon-Herb Dressing from the Kind Kale Salad (page 199) for the Tzatziki Dressing and substituting plain Marvelous Macadamia Cheese (page 219) for the Fanciful Feta Cheese or omitting it altogether.

Serves 1 or 2, with leftover dressing

Tzatziki Dressing

(Makes about 2 cups/470 milliliters)

1½ cups (350 milliliters) Cashew Yogurt (recipe follows)

4 teaspoons fresh lemon juice

2 teaspoons extra-virgin olive oil

1 garlic clove, pressed through a garlic press or grated

2 tablespoons finely chopped dill

1 teaspoon grated lemon zest

¾ teaspoon salt

Pinch of freshly ground black pepper

½ cup (70 grams) shredded cucumber (about ½ small cucumber)

Salad

3 cups (about 70 grams) torn romaine lettuce leaves

1 plum tomato, chopped

½ red bell pepper, cored, seeded, and chopped

½ cucumber, end trimmed and chopped

1 scallion, chopped

Handful of kalamata olives, pitted

Handful of capers

4 to 6 pieces Fanciful Feta Cheese (page 222)

[195]

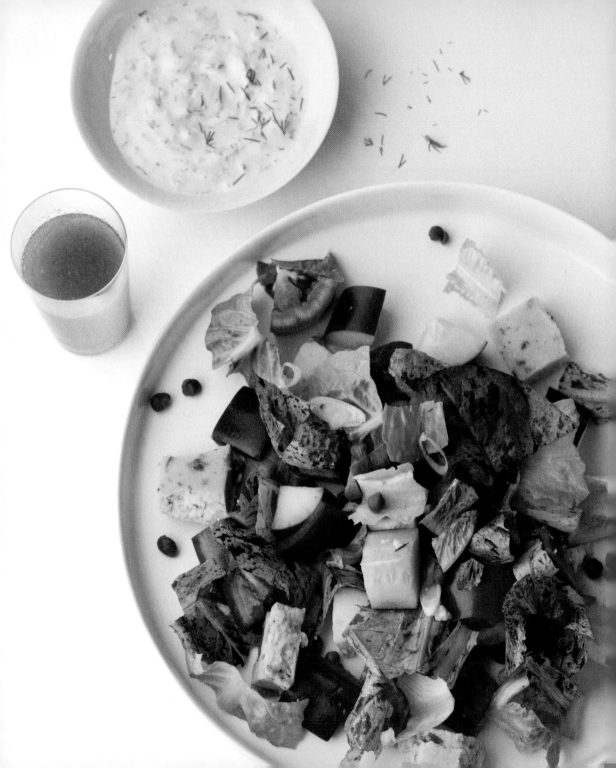

Make the Tzatziki Dressing: Whisk together all the ingredients except the cucumber in a medium bowl. Stir in the cucumber.

Make the salad: Combine all the ingredients except the feta cheese in a salad bowl and toss to combine. Add dressing to taste and toss to coat. Top with the feta cheese and serve immediately. Pour the remaining dressing into a covered container and store refrigerated for up to 5 days.

Cashew Yogurt
Makes about 2 cups (470 milliliters)

2 cups (225 grams) cashews, soaked in water to cover overnight and drained
1½ cups (350 milliliters) water
1½ teaspoons acidophilus powder

In a food processor or high-speed blender, combine the cashews, water, and acidophilus powder and blend until very smooth, about 5 minutes, stopping the machine every so often to scrape down the sides and resting it to keep the mixture from getting too warm.

[197]

Transfer the mixture to a stainless-steel or glass container, cover tightly with plastic wrap, and leave in a warm part of the kitchen (like on top of the refrigerator) to ferment for 12 hours. To speed up the process, ferment the cheese in a dehydrator set to 90°F (32°C). The yogurt will keep refrigerated for up to 2 weeks.

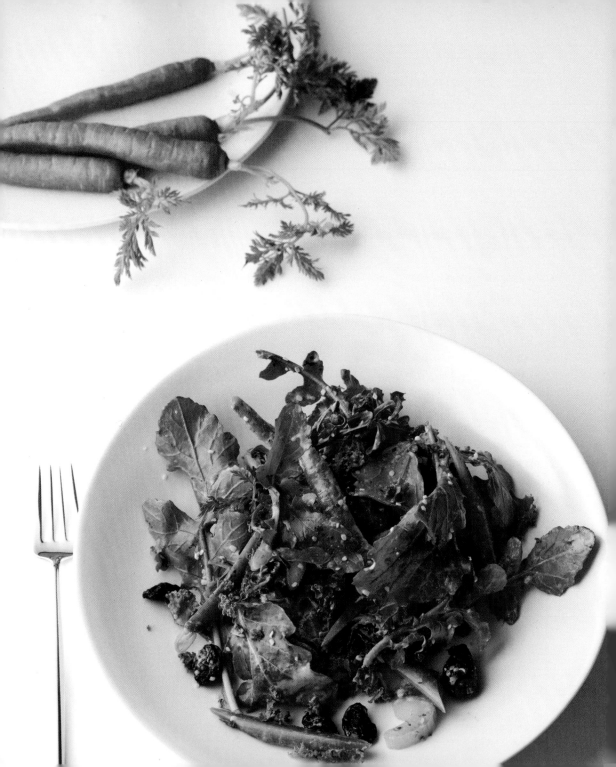

Kind Kale Salad with Lemon-Herb Dressing

This salad is a LOVE* staple: The play of bitter, salty, and sweet from the kale, olives, and raisins is at once a surprise and a delight, and it keeps people coming back for more.

Serves 1 or 2, with leftover dressing

Lemon-Herb Dressing

(Makes about 1 cup/240 milliliters)

⅓ cup (70 milliliters) fresh lemon juice, or more to taste

1 date, soaked in water to cover for 2 to 3 hours, drained, and pitted

1 garlic clove, cut in half

½ teaspoon dried thyme

½ teaspoon dried oregano

¼ teaspoon salt, or more to taste

Pinch of freshly ground black pepper

⅔ cup (140 milliliters) extra-virgin olive oil

Salad

1½ cups (about 35 grams) torn or shredded kale leaves

1½ cups (25 grams) baby arugula

1 small carrot, shredded, or a few slender young carrots

½ small celery stalk, chopped

Handful of kalamata olives, pitted

Handful of raisins

1 teaspoon hemp seeds

[199]

Make the Lemon-Herb Dressing: Combine all the ingredients except the oil in a blender and blend until combined. With the motor running, drizzle the oil in through the hole in the top until the dressing is emulsified. Taste and adjust the seasonings with lemon juice and salt if needed.

Make the salad: Combine all the ingredients except the hemp seeds in a salad bowl and toss to combine. Add dressing to taste and toss to coat. Top with the hemp seeds and serve immediately. Pour the remaining dressing into a covered container and store refrigerated for up to 5 days.

DID YOU KNOW?
Per calorie, kale has more iron than beef and more calcium than dairy milk.

Amazing Arugula Salad with Caring Carrot Cheese and Caesar Dressing

Arugula is a cruciferous veggie that is loaded with free radical–fighting phyto-chemicals and is a good source of calcium; iron; manganese; copper; potassium; vitamins A, C, K; and folic acid. The crowning touch is Organic Avenue's signature carrot cheese, a recipe our customers have been asking for since we first introduced it to our menu.

Serves 1 or 2, with leftover dressing

Caesar Dressing

(Makes about ¾ cup/175 milliliters)

¼ cup (60 milliliters) water
⅓ cup (70 milliliters) extra-virgin olive oil
1 garlic clove, cut in half
1 large celery stalk, chopped
2 tablespoons fresh lemon juice, or more
    to taste
1 teaspoon white chickpea miso
1 date, soaked in water to cover for
    2 to 3 hours, drained, and pitted
1 teaspoon tamari
¼ teaspoon salt, or more to taste
Pinch of freshly ground black pepper, or
    more to taste

Salad

3 cups (50 grams) baby arugula leaves
Handful of sunflower sprouts
½ red bell pepper, cored, seeded, and
    cut into thin strips
1 sun-dried tomato, soaked in water
    to cover for 2 to 3 hours, drained,
    patted dry, and cut into slivers
Handful of walnut halves
6 to 8 squares Caring Carrot Cheese
    (page 220)

Make the Caesar Dressing: Combine all the ingredients except the oil in a blender and blend until smooth. With the motor running, drizzle the oil in through the hole in the top until the dressing is emulsified. Taste and adjust the seasonings with lemon juice, salt, and pepper if needed.

Make the salad: Combine the arugula, sunflower sprouts, bell pepper, and sun-dried tomato in a salad bowl and toss to combine. Add dressing to taste and

[200]

toss to coat. Top with the walnuts and carrot cheese. Serve immediately. Pour the remaining dressing into a covered container and store refrigerated for up to 5 days.

SWEET NATURE FROM NATURE

Lately in some circles the carrot has gotten a bad rap for its sweet nature. My take on the subject: Its sweet nature is *from* nature. And as I live on a plant-based diet, I don't like to exclude any fruit, vegetable, nut, seed, or seaweed, as long as it's not poisonous. Cutting out a carrot would be like cutting out the color orange from the rainbow! And, interesting enough, if you chew on a carrot, it can help to reduce bacteria in your mouth and clean your teeth.

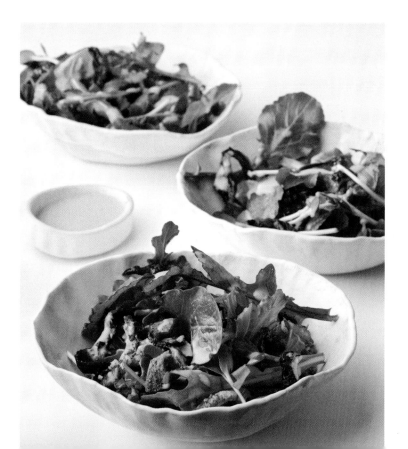

Sun-Kissed Kale and Collard Salad with Coconut-Miso Dressing

Here the almighty kale partners with collard greens to deliver a double dose of cancer-preventative compounds. Quinoa provides a nice balance of amino acids, and to finish, the salad is bathed in a heavenly coconut-creamy miso-flavored dressing. If you're looking to get close to 100 percent raw (or already are!), substitute sprouted quinoa for the cooked, and if you don't have time to make the Spicy Pumpkin Seeds, simple raw pumpkin seeds are perfectly fine.

Serves 1 or 2, with leftover dressing

[202]

Coconut-Miso Dressing
(Makes about 1 cup/240 milliliters)

¼ cup (60 milliliters) water

2 tablespoons coconut water

¼ cup (15 grams) packed fresh coconut meat (see page 146)

1½ tablespoons fresh lime juice, or more to taste

1 tablespoon shredded dried coconut

1 tablespoon white chickpea miso

1 teaspoon coconut sugar

½ teaspoon salt, or more to taste

Pinch of freshly ground black pepper, or more to taste

¼ cup (60 milliliters) extra-virgin olive oil

Salad

3 cups (about 70 grams) mixed kale and collard green leaves cut into ribbons or shredded (see Note)

¼ cup (45 grams) cooked red or tan quinoa (or substitute sprouted quinoa to keep it all raw)

2 tablespoons Spicy Pumpkin Seeds (page 275)

1 tablespoon shredded dried coconut

Make the Coconut-Miso Dressing: Combine all the ingredients except the oil in a blender and blend until combined. With the motor running, drizzle the oil in through the hole in the top until the dressing is emulsified. Taste and adjust the seasonings with lime juice, salt, and pepper if needed.

Make the salad: Combine all the ingredients in a salad bowl and toss to combine. Add dressing to taste and toss to coat. Serve immediately. Pour the remaining dressing into a covered container and store refrigerated for up to 5 days.

> **NOTE**
> To shred kale, roughly tear the leaves and pulse them in a food processor until shredded to your liking.

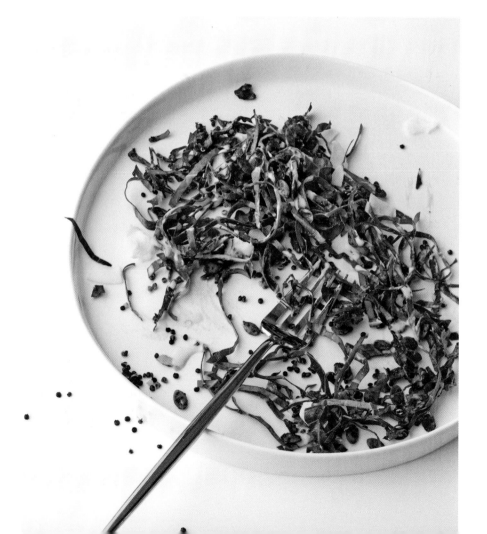

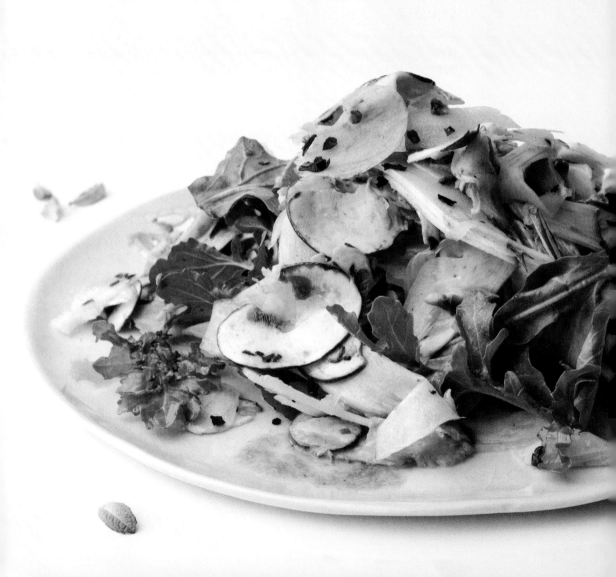

Mighty Mushroom and Fennel Salad with Arugula and Lemon-Mint Dressing

Mushrooms provide magical nutrient density to this salad. The selenium found in most varieties of mushrooms gives weight loss a mighty boost, and their anti-oxidant properties will work against aging and help out your immune system. In case you'd like more reasons to LOVE* mushrooms, the selenium content provides healthy protection to the bladder and prostate. A generous amount of arugula to finish the salad has you covered in the green department.

Serves 1 or 2, with leftover dressing

Lemon-Mint Dressing
(Makes just under 1 cup/210 milliliters)

¼ cup (60 milliliters) fresh lemon juice, or more to taste

¼ cup (15 grams) mint leaves

¼ teaspoon salt, or more to taste

Pinch of freshly ground black pepper, or more to taste

10 tablespoons (150 milliliters) extra-virgin olive oil

Salad
¾ cup (150 grams) marinated mushrooms (page 262)

¼ cup (15 grams) shaved fennel

2 cups (40 grams) baby arugula leaves

[205]

Make the Lemon-Mint Dressing: Combine all the ingredients except the oil in a blender and blend until the mint is blended in. With the motor running, drizzle the oil in through the hole in the top until the dressing is emulsified. Taste and adjust the seasonings with lemon juice, salt, and pepper if needed.

Make the salad: Combine the mushrooms and fennel in a salad bowl and toss to combine. Toss in the arugula, then add dressing to taste and toss to coat. Serve immediately. Pour the remaining dressing into a covered container and store refrigerated for up to 5 days.

Calming Cauliflower Salad

Cauliflower is a member of the cruciferous family, which is known for its cancer-fighting properties, and when you eat any crucifer *raw*, those properties are even more pronounced. For those of us unaccustomed to eating cauliflower in the raw, the secret to making it both raw and delicious is to slice it very thinly or chop it finely, then marinate it with oil, citrus, and spices. We fancy up our cauliflower salad with an unconventional combination of mint, dates, turmeric, cayenne, and cacao nibs, and, put simply, it works. Our customers will attest to it!

Serves 4 as a side dish

1 medium head cauliflower, very thinly sliced or finely chopped
¼ cup (30 grams) finely chopped cashews
3 dates, soaked in water to cover for 2 to 3 hours, drained, pitted, and finely
  chopped
3 tablespoons liquid coconut oil
2 tablespoons fresh lemon juice
½ teaspoon ground turmeric
½ teaspoon salt
¼ teaspoon freshly ground black pepper
Pinch of ground cayenne
¼ cup (7 grams) chopped cilantro leaves
¼ cup (7 grams) chopped mint leaves
2 tablespoons cacao nibs

In a large bowl, combine the cauliflower, cashews, and dates.

In a small bowl, whisk together the oil, lemon juice, turmeric, salt, pepper, and cayenne. Add it to the cauliflower mixture and toss to coat very well. Add the cilantro, mint, and cacao nibs and toss to coat. Serve immediately, or place in a container, cover, and refrigerate until ready to serve. It will keep for 3 to 4 days.

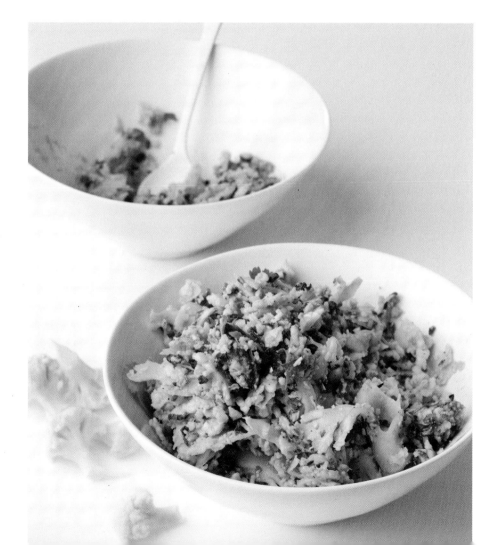

[207]

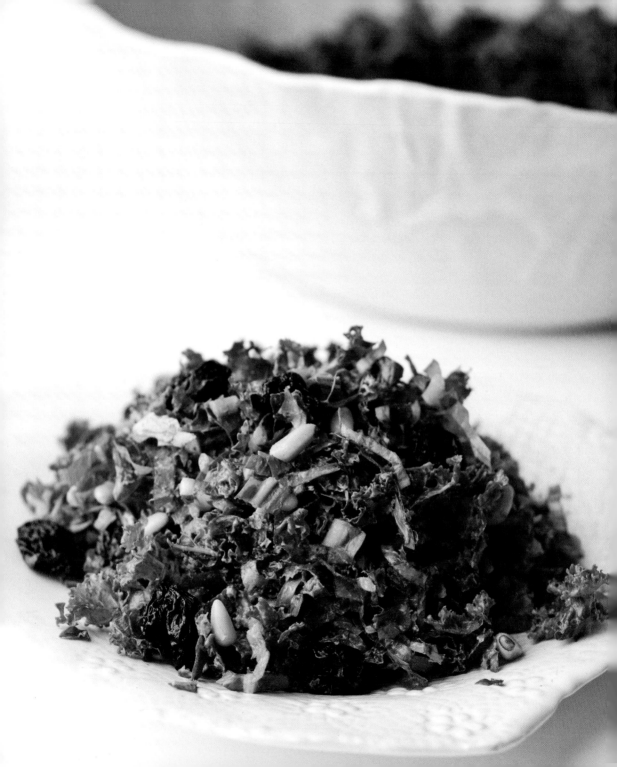

Delicious Dandelion Salad with Ranch Dressing

Bitter is a taste largely overlooked in the standard American diet, which may in part explain our addiction to sugary junk foods. Bitter expands the palate and offsets the more familiar flavors of salty and sweet, and the bitterness in dandelion greens, for example, assists the liver in detoxification, which makes this salad a good one to turn to when you're cleansing.

Further benefits of dandelion include relief from diabetes, urinary disorders, acne, jaundice, inflammation, and anemia. Dandelion also helps in maintaining bone health, skin care, and weight loss. Enough said?

Serves 4 as a side dish, with leftover dressing

Ranch Dressing
(Makes about 1¼ cups/300 milliliters)

½ cup (120 milliliters) water
½ cup (60 grams) hemp seeds
½ cup (65 grams) pine nuts
2 garlic cloves, cut in half
2½ tablespoons fresh lemon juice, or more to taste
Small section of jalapeño chile, or to taste, seeded
½ teaspoon salt, or more to taste
Pinch of freshly ground black pepper
¼ cup (60 milliliters) extra-virgin olive oil
¾ teaspoon dried dill

Salad

2 cups (about 45 grams) shredded kale leaves (see Note, page 203)
1 cup (about 20 grams) torn dandelion leaves
2 tablespoons raisins
2 tablespoons pine nuts

[209]

Make the Ranch Dressing: Combine all the ingredients except the oil and dill in a blender and blend until smooth. With the motor running, drizzle the oil in through the hole in the top until the dressing is emulsified. Add the dill and blend to combine. Taste and adjust the seasonings with lemon juice and salt if needed.

Make the salad: Combine the kale and dandelion leaves in a salad bowl and toss to combine. Add dressing to taste and toss to coat. Taste and adjust the seasonings if needed. Top with the raisins and pine nuts. Serve immediately, or cover and refrigerate until ready to serve. Pour the remaining dressing into a covered container and store refrigerated for up to 5 days.

DID YOU KNOW?

If you're growing dandelion greens in your garden or foraging them from a field, make sure to use the leaves when they are young; full-grown dandelion leaves can be overpoweringly bitter.

Blessed Beet Salad with Preserved Lemon–Mint Dressing

Beets are a lifesaver. The pigment that gives them their crimson color, beta-cyanin, is a powerful cancer-fighting agent, particularly effective against colon cancer according to some studies. Other lifesaving properties of beets: they contain ample magnesium, calcium, iron, and phosphorus, not to mention the fiber that keeps things moving. Carrots also may help prevent colon cancer as well as detox the liver and blood, slow down the aging of cells, and treat acne and even out skin tone.

Here these two sweet root vegetables are shredded, then treated to a slightly tart, intensely citrusy dressing featuring preserved lemon, a naturally fermented condiment often used in North African cuisine; it can be found in Middle Eastern groceries or international food stores.

Serves 4 as a side dish, with leftover dressing

Preserved Lemon–Mint Dressing

(Makes about 1 cup/240 milliliters)

½ cup (120 milliliters) water
¼ cup (15 grams) mint leaves
2 garlic cloves, cut in half
1 tablespoon fresh lemon juice, or more to
   taste
½ preserved lemon, chopped
½ cup (120 milliliters) extra-virgin olive oil
Salt if needed

Salad

4 carrots, coarsely shredded
2 medium beets, peeled and
   coarsely shredded
Handful of pistachios

Make the Preserved Lemon–Mint Dressing: Combine all the ingredients except the oil in a blender and blend until smooth. With the motor running, drizzle the oil in through the hole in the top until the dressing is emulsified. Taste and adjust the seasonings with lemon juice and salt if needed.

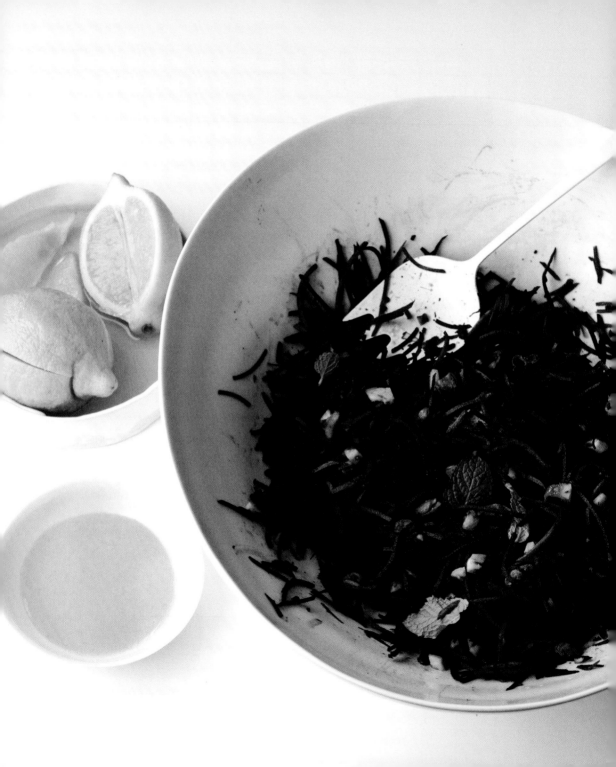

Make the salad: Combine the carrots and beets in a salad bowl and toss to combine. Add dressing to taste and toss to coat. Taste and adjust the seasonings if needed. Top with the pistachios and serve immediately, or cover and refrigerate until ready to serve. Pour the remaining dressing into a covered container and store refrigerated for up to 5 days.

[213]

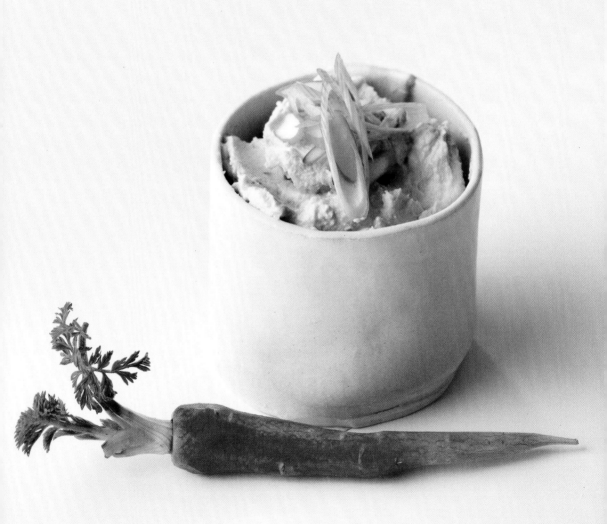

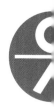

Cheeses, Dips, and Spreads

The *New York Times* named fermentation as one of the top ten food trends of 2013. Many of us are familiar with everyday fermented foods such as sauerkraut, pickles, and the like, but at Organic Avenue, we do something a little different: We ferment nuts—cashews and macadamias—to make our vegan cheeses, employing acidophilus to provide a probiotic punch. Our cashew and macadamia cheeses are for spreading, our feta and carrot cheeses are welcome toppers to our salads, and the pine nut Parm gives our noodle dishes an Italian-inspired accent. Our hummus, guacamole, and Lebanese dip complete the profile, providing you with an assortment of crudité accompaniments, sandwich fillings, and chip-scoopable treats.

[215]

Opposite: Confident Cashew Cream Cheese (page 216)

Confident Cashew Cream Cheese

This creamy spreadable cheese, made from blending cashews and culturing them with acidophilus powder, is often mistaken for dairy cheese, infinitely satisfying both the lactose intolerant and vegans among us. Make sure you blend your cashews very well, with a goal of a smooth cream cheese–like texture; this can take up to five minutes.

This recipe makes a generous quantity; this is because the blender needs a good amount of volume to complete its magical transformation of cashews into cheese. Fortunately, the final product keeps for up to two weeks, though its seductive spreadability most likely will cause it to disappear much sooner. Feel free to substitute other herbs or spices for the scallions—mix and match and see what you like.

Makes about 3 cups (650 grams)

4 cups (1 pound/450 grams) raw cashews, soaked in water to cover for 8 hours
   or overnight and drained
¾ cup (180 ml) water
1 tablespoon acidophilus powder (see Note)
1 tablespoon onion powder
1½ teaspoons salt
4 scallions, white and green parts, minced

In a high-speed blender, combine the cashews, water, and acidophilus powder and blend until very smooth, about 5 minutes, stopping the machine every so often to scrape down the sides and resting it to keep the mixture from getting too warm.

Transfer the mixture to a stainless-steel or glass container, cover tightly with plastic wrap, and leave in a warm part of the kitchen (like on top of the refrigerator or the dehydrator if you've got it going) to ferment for 12 hours.

The next day, stir in the onion powder and salt, then fold in the scallions. The cheese will keep, covered and refrigerated, for up to 2 weeks.

NOTE

Acidophilus powder can be found in the refrigerated area of your natural food store's supplement section. Make sure you choose a brand labeled "dairy-free."

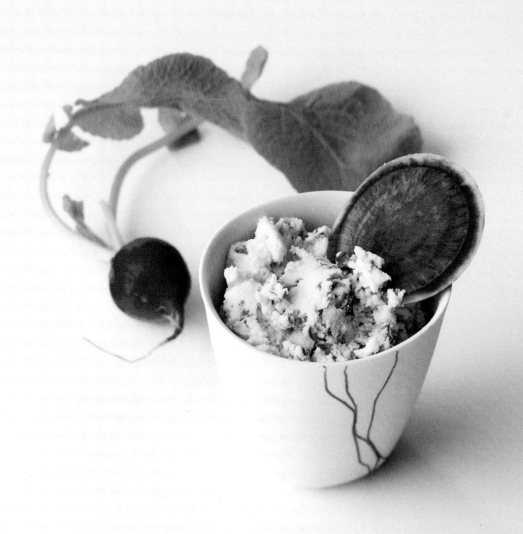

Marvelous Macadamia Cheese

Somewhat like farmer cheese in texture and taste and the base for our Fanciful Feta Cheese (page 222), this cheese, like our Confident Cashew Cream Cheese (page 216), is fermented with acidophilus to a state of extreme nutrition and savory deliciousness. Macadamias are magnificently medicinal, high in B-complex vitamins, vitamins A and E, calcium, iron, magnesium, manganese, and zinc. These little creations are here to serve your good health. Trust me. Eat this cheese. Regularly!

Makes about 3 cups (650 grams)

4 cups (1 pound/450 grams) macadamia nuts
1¾ cups (420 milliliters) water
1 tablespoon acidophilus powder (see Note, page 217)
1 tablespoon onion powder
1½ teaspoons salt
¼ cup (30 grams) minced parsley, chives, or other fresh herb

In a high-speed blender, combine the macadamias, water, and acidophilus powder and blend until very smooth, about 5 minutes, stopping the machine every so often to scrape down the sides and resting it to keep the mixture from getting too warm.

[219]

Transfer the mixture to a stainless-steel or glass container, cover tightly with plastic wrap, and leave in a warm part of the kitchen (like on top of the refrigerator or the dehydrator if you've got it going) to ferment for 12 hours.

The next day, remove the extra liquid from the mixture by squeezing it through a nut milk bag or double layer of cheesecloth. Return to the bowl, stir in the onion powder and salt, then mix in the herbs. The cheese will keep, covered and refrigerated, for up to 2 weeks.

Caring Carrot Cheese

Our customers asked for it, and here it is: our signature carrot cheese, familiar as the crowning touch of our Amazing Arugula Salad (page 200), though it could be served with any salad in this book or of your own creation, on crackers, or with cocktail sticks as a passed hors d'oeuvre. While this recipe isn't difficult, it does involve several steps, first of which is saving the pulp from your carrot juice and then dehydrating it. Plan your carrot cheese in advance; you'll find it's worth the extra effort.

Makes about thirty-six 1-inch (2.5-centimeter) cheese squares

⅔ cup (5 ounces/140 grams) Confident Cashew Cream Cheese (page 216)
½ cup (3 ounces/85 grams) Marvelous Macadamia Cheese (page 219)
2 tablespoons white chickpea miso
¼ cup (40 grams) Carrot Powder (recipe follows)

In a medium bowl, combine all the ingredients. Mix well, starting with a fork to incorporate the ingredients and then kneading with your hands a few times to fully blend. Form the mixture into an approximately 6-inch (15-centimeter) square that is ½ inch (1.25 centimeters) thick onto a ParaFlexx-lined dehydrator sheet. Set the dehydrator to 110°F (40°C) and dehydrate for 1 hour, or until a light crust starts to form on the outside but the inside is still quite soft. Flip the cheese directly onto a mesh dehydrator screen and dehydrate for another hour, or until a crust forms on the second side with the inside remaining soft. Cut into 1-inch (2.5-centimeter) squares. Store, covered and refrigerated, for up to 2 weeks.

" Leave good things alone. Work on the blatant and bad. Later you can work on making the good things great."

—DENISE MARI

Carrot Powder

Instead of composting the pulp from your carrot juice, use it to make this carrot powder. It conveniently calls for the amount of carrots required to make 16 ounces of Caring Carrot Juice (page 117). If you're a frequent carrot juicer, save your pulp and make a big batch of the powder, which also doubles as a sprinkle for salads, soups, or wherever you'd like a slightly sweet, highly nutritious flavor accent.

About 3 cups (10 ounces/300 grams) carrot pulp (from juicing about 2 pounds
   carrots; page 117)

Spread the carrot pulp onto a ParaFlexx-lined dehydrator sheet. Set the dehydrator to 110°F (40°C) and dehydrate for about 5 hours, until the pulp is completely dry. Transfer to a high-speed blender or spice grinder and blend until the pulp breaks down into powder.

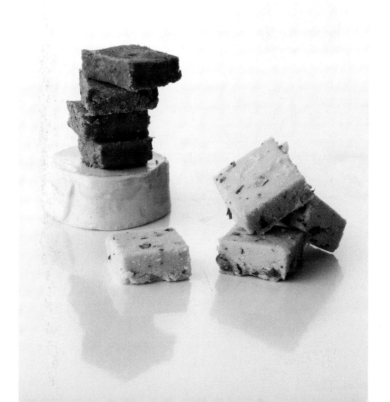

Fanciful Feta Cheese

This cheese was originally created for our Big Greek Salad (page 195), but it makes a smart cheese topping for any salad, or you could spread it on crackers or inside a collard leaf wrap. It requires a bit of work—making two separate cheeses—but as a timsaver you might consider making it with just the Marvelous Macadamia Cheese, which will result in a feta that is slightly less creamy and more crumbly but equally tasty.

Makes about 36 1-inch (2.5-centimeter) cheese squares

1 cup (6 ounces/170 grams) Marvelous Macadamia Cheese (page 219)
¾ cup (6 ounces/170 grams) Confident Cashew Cream Cheese (page 216)
½ cup (55 grams) coconut flour
1½ tablespoons white chickpea miso

In a medium bowl, combine all the ingredients. Mix well, starting with a fork to incorporate the ingredients and then kneading with your hands a few times to fully blend. Form the mixture into an approximately 6-inch (15-centimeter) square that is ½ inch (1.25 centimeters) thick onto a ParaFlexx-lined dehydrator sheet. Set the dehydrator to 110°F (40°C) and dehydrate for 1 hour, or until a light crust starts to form on the outside but the inside is still quite soft. Flip the cheese directly onto a mesh dehydrator screen and dehydrate for another hour, or until a crust forms on the second side with the inside remaining soft. Cut into 1-inch (2.5-centimeter) squares or, alternatively, loosely crumble the cheese. Store, covered and refrigerated, for up to 2 weeks.

Plentiful Pine Nut Parmesan

Another way to add culture to your cheese plate: fermenting pine nuts with acidophilus and dehydrating to a state of Parmesan crispness is sure to delight and amaze those not partaking in dairy cheese (and even those who are!). Sprinkle on soups, salads, pasta dishes—anywhere you'd use traditional Parm.

Makes about 4 cups cheese shavings (260 grams)

2 cups (260 grams) pine nuts
1¼ cups (300 milliliters) water
½ teaspoon acidophilus powder (see Note, page 217)
1½ teaspoons salt

In a high-speed blender, combine the pine nuts, water, and acidophilus powder and blend until very smooth, about 5 minutes, stopping the machine every so often to scrape down the sides and resting it to keep the mixture from getting too warm.

Transfer the mixture to a stainless-steel or glass container, cover tightly with plastic wrap, and leave in a warm part of the kitchen (like on top of the refrigerator or the dehydrator if you've got it going) to ferment for 12 hours.

The next day, stir in the salt. Spread a thin layer of the mixture (as thin as you can get without it becoming translucent) over ParaFlexx-lined dehydrator sheets. Set the dehydrator to 110°F (40°C) and dehydrate for about 24 hours, until completely dry and crisp. Pull the cheese from the sheets and break into pieces. Store in an airtight container at room temperature for up to 2 months.

[223]

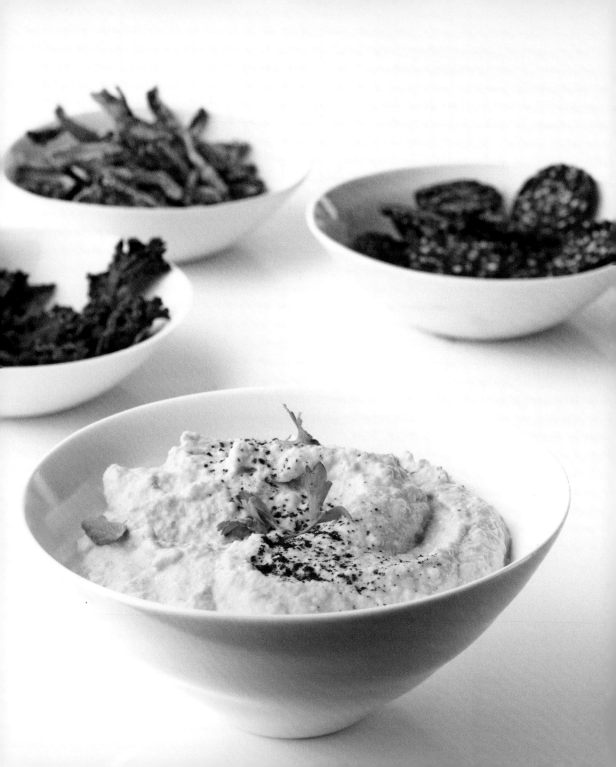

Happy Hummus

Who says hummus has to be made with chickpeas? If you're keeping close to the LOVE*Lifestyle, try Organic Avenue's take on the dip, based on sesame seeds and zucchini and totally raw. Think of zucchini as a blank slate: neutral in flavor and just waiting for you to fancy it up, whether as noodles (see pages 258 to 265) or here by blending it with the familiar hummus ingredients tahini and lemon juice.

Makes about 3 cups (650 grams)

1 small to medium zucchini (about 8 ounces/220 grams), chopped
1 cup (5 ounces/140 grams) sunflower seeds, soaked in water to cover overnight
   and drained
½ cup (120 milliliters) tahini
¼ cup (60 milliliters) fresh lemon juice
2 tablespoons extra-virgin olive oil
1 garlic clove, cut in half
1 teaspoon salt
¼ teaspoon ground cayenne
Garnishes: extra-virgin olive oil, black olive slices, chopped parsley, paprika

[225]

Combine all the ingredients except the garnishes in a food processor or high-speed blender and process until silky smooth, stopping to scrape the sides as needed and to cool the machine; this may take up to 5 minutes. Serve with the garnishes, with crudités or crackers alongside. The hummus will keep, covered and refrigerated, for up to 5 days.

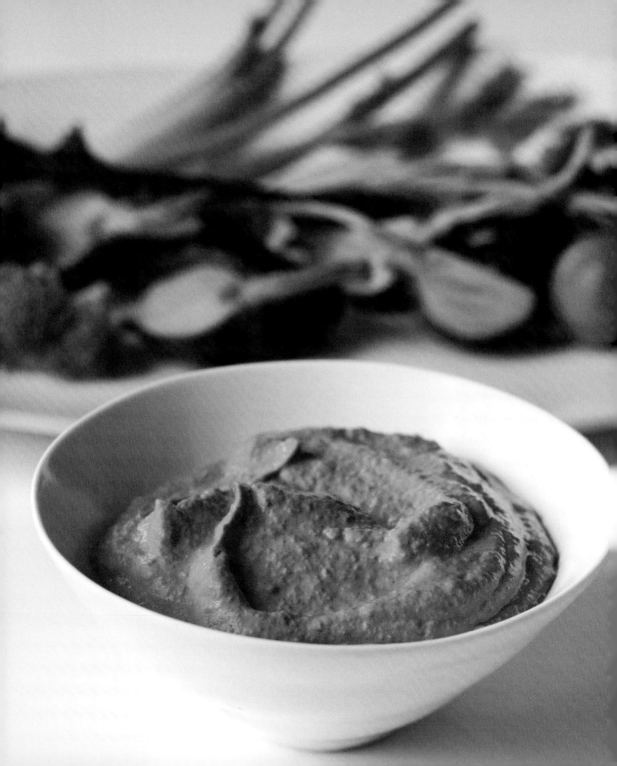

Lucky Lebanese Dip

Just the right combination of flavorings, seasonings, and herbs makes me feel lucky every time I dip a carrot into this Middle Eastern–style tahini-based dip. It's also what we serve our falafel (page 255) with.

Makes just under 1 cup (220 grams)

¼ cup (60 milliliters) fresh lemon juice
⅓ cup (2½ ounces/75 grams) tahini
¼ cup (60 milliliters) extra-virgin olive oil
1 tablespoon water
1 garlic clove, cut in half
¼ teaspoon salt
Pinch of freshly ground black pepper
Pinch of ground cayenne
1½ tablespoons thinly sliced scallion
1½ tablespoons minced parsley

Combine the lemon juice, tahini, oil, water, garlic, salt, and peppers in a blender and blend until smooth. Pour into a bowl, add the scallion and parsley, and stir to combine. Store in the refrigerator in an airtight container for up to 5 days.

[227]

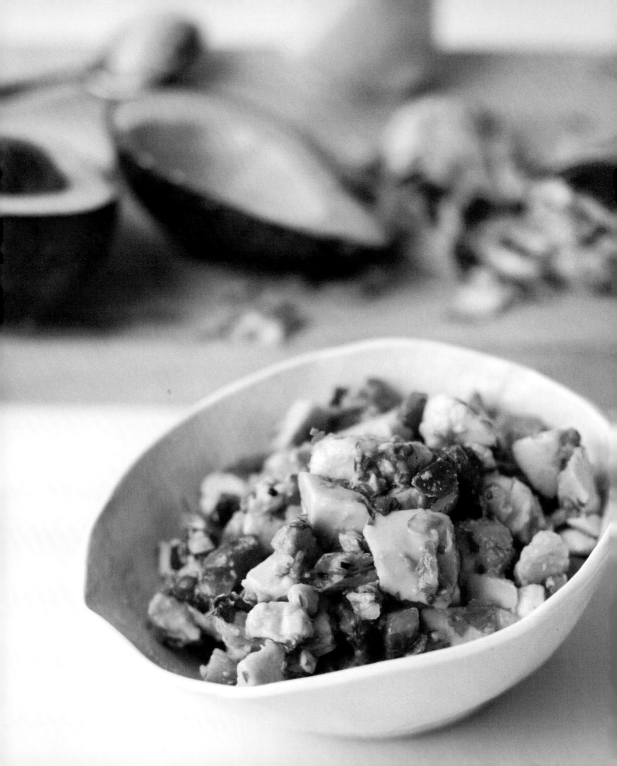

Guapo Guacamole

The classic, from sixteenth-century Aztec Mexico to Super Bowl Sunday. Scale up accordingly for the latter.

Makes about 1½ cups (350 grams)

3 medium ripe avocados (about 1 pound/450 grams)
1 medium plum tomato (about 5 ounces/140 grams), cored, seeded, and diced
1 tablespoon chopped cilantro
1 tablespoon fresh lime juice, or more to taste
2 tablespoons minced red onion
¼ teaspoon ground cumin
½ teaspoon salt
Pinch of freshly ground black pepper
Pinch of ground cayenne

Cut the avocados in half, remove the pits, and scoop the flesh into a large bowl. Smash it with a fork—a lot if you like your guacamole smooth, a little if you like it chunky. Add the remaining ingredients, mix well, and serve, with crudités, crackers, or chips, or place a scoop atop the salad of your choice.

[229]

FEAR NOT FAT

Don't be scared of our fatty friend the avocado, because avocado contains good, monounsaturated fat, and good fats replace bad fats and release the pleasure sensors in the brain. We want these good fats because they're what our cell membrane is made of, and our brains are a good percentage fat.

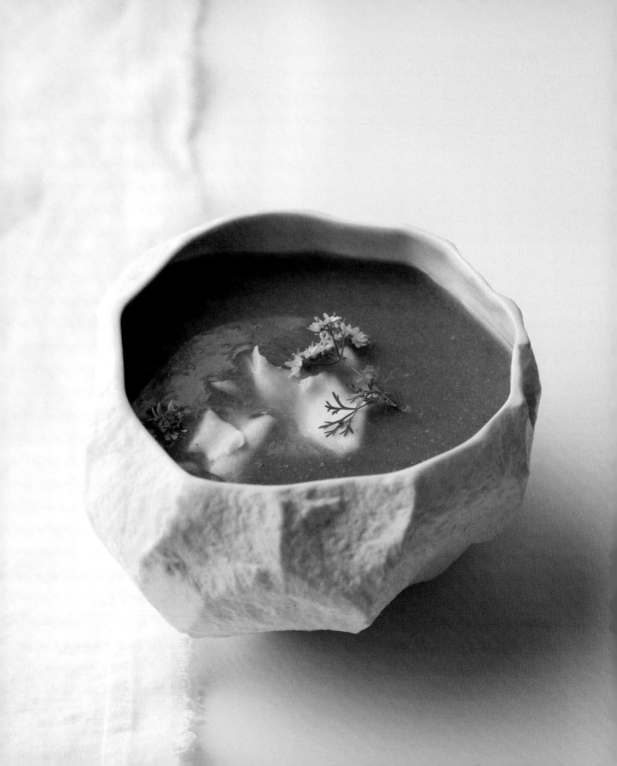

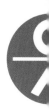

Soups

LOVE* soups are made start to finish right in the blender, no pots and pans required, leaving minimal cleanup at the end of the meal. What could be more appealing on a hot summer day? Or in cooler temps, run the blender a little longer to warm the soup, *warm* being the operative word, as you can literally cook your soup if the blender runs too long, especially if you are using a high-speed blender, our tool of choice for silky-smooth Organic Avenue soups (see page 55 for more on this type of blender). This way you'll get the comfort of a cooked soup while keeping your commitment to raw.

Organic Avenue soups are a staple in the LOVE*Lifestyle, both as everyday dishes and specific cleanse items (see page 67 for the LOVE*Cleanse menus). An all-liquid diet for a period of time can provide tremendous healing for the body; while juices offer a complete digestive break, soups provide a rest from solid food but still give us the natural fiber that we need to keep things going. For many people, particularly those of us with a busy lifestyle, including a substantial soup in our cleanse routine gives us the sustenance to go the distance while going about our daily routine.

These four top Organic Avenue living soups get their blender-to-bowl deliciousness from fresh ingredients and bold flavors rather than time spent on a stovetop. They include tomatoes, both fresh and sun-dried; coconut and avocado, to provide a creamy base minus the cream; and citrus, herbs, and spices, to bring the flavors together to please the palate any time of year, any time of day.

Opposite: Tasty Thai Coconut Soup (page 238)

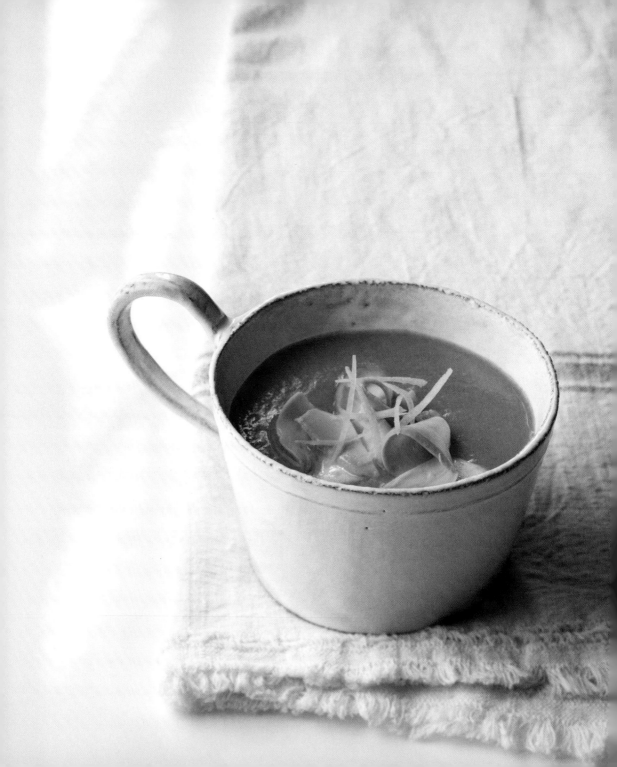

Awesome Avocado Mint Soup

Think guacamole in a glass, oh-so-satisfying as a light summer meal or a more substantial one when paired with one of our salad offerings (pages 195 to 213). Avocados are rich in luteins and folate, both important for heart health, and spinach and mint pump up the green factor, always a good thing in the LOVE*Lifestyle.

Serves 2 to 4 (makes about 4 cups/1 liter)

2½ cups (600 milliliters) water
1 small avocado, peeled and pitted
1 small unpeeled cucumber, ends trimmed and roughly chopped
½ cup (15 grams) packed mint leaves
Handful of spinach leaves
1 garlic clove, cut in half
2 tablespoons fresh lime juice, or more to taste
1¼ teaspoons salt, or more to taste
¼ teaspoon freshly ground black pepper

[233]

Combine all the ingredients in a high-speed blender and blend until smooth, adding more water if the soup is too thick. Taste and adjust the seasonings with salt and lime juice if needed. Serve immediately, or cover and keep in the refrigerator until ready to serve.

DID YOU KNOW?
Avocados are high in beta sitosterol, a compound that has been shown to lower LDL ("bad") cholesterol levels. Another reason to include avocados in a heart-healthy diet.

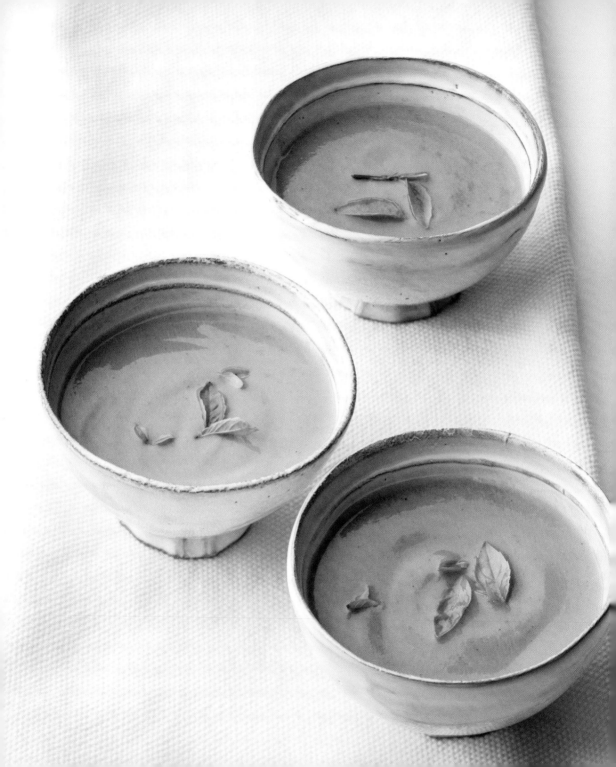

Terrific Tomato Basil Soup

Nothing says summer quite like a juicy farmers'-market tomato. But what to do when tomato season is over and all that's available is a selection of nowhere-close-to-local pale and sad-looking tomatoes? Blend up a batch of this soup, which features sun-dried tomatoes, available 365 days a year.

Serves 2 to 4 (makes about 4 cups/1 liter)

1 small avocado, peeled and pitted
1 tablespoon fresh lime juice, or more to taste
½ cup (30 grams) sun-dried tomatoes, soaked in water to cover for 2 to 3 hours
    and drained
3 cups (700 ml) water
1 scallion, white and green parts, chopped
⅓ cup (10 grams) basil leaves, roughly chopped
1 or 2 garlic cloves, cut in half
1½ teaspoons salt, or more to taste
¼ cup freshly ground black pepper
Pinch of ground cayenne

[235]

Combine all the ingredients in a high-speed blender and blend until smooth, adding more water if the soup is too thick. Taste and adjust the seasonings with salt and lime juice if needed. Serve immediately, or cover and keep in the refrigerator until ready to serve.

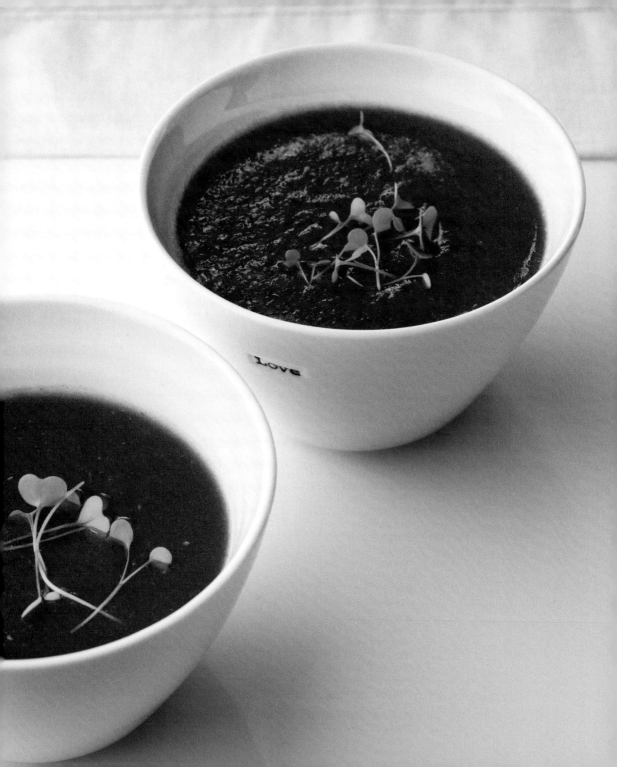

Totally Tomato and Tarragon Soup

Tarragon, with its distinctive licorice flavor, makes a clear flavor statement in this lively, slightly spicy tomato-based soup. This herb is considered one of the finest spices in French cooking, but while it appeals to the sophisticated palate, let's not overlook its many healing properties, including its use as an antioxidant, digestive aid, and cardiovascular health promoter. Favor fresh tarragon, as the flavor will be more intense and the healing benefits more pronounced, but in a pinch 1 teaspoon dried tarragon can stand in.

Serves 2 to 4 (makes about 4 cups/1 liter)

1½ cups (350 milliliters) water
3 medium fresh tomatoes (about 14 ounces/400 grams), chopped
⅓ cup (15 grams) sun-dried tomatoes, soaked in water for 2 to 3 hours, drained, and chopped
1 tablespoon fresh tarragon leaves or 1 teaspoon dried tarragon
2 tablespoons fresh lemon juice, or more to taste
¼ small jalapeño chile, seeded and minced, or to taste
1 garlic clove, cut in half
1 teaspoon salt, or more to taste

[237]

Combine all the ingredients in a high-speed blender and blend until smooth, adding more water if the soup is too thick. Taste and adjust the seasonings with salt and lemon juice if needed. Serve immediately, or cover and keep in the refrigerator until ready to serve.

❝ We all need to eat, but blending food helps us to do what we all tend to do less than perfectly: chew!"

—DENISE MARI

Tasty Thai Coconut Soup

Oh, how we love the versatility of the coconut, in our smoothies, in desserts, and in this soup, where its water provides the base and the meat its creaminess; together they welcome the familiar palette of Asian spices that we have all come to know and love.

Serves 2 to 4 (makes about 4 cups/1 liter)

1 cup (240 milliliters) water

1 cup (240 milliliters) Clearly Coconut Water (page 145) or bottled raw coconut water

2 cups (12 ounces/340 grams) packed fresh coconut meat (see page 146)

1 garlic clove, cut in half

Small piece of jalapeño chile, seeded, or to taste

1 tablespoon fresh lime juice, or more to taste

½ teaspoon ground coriander

½ teaspoon curry powder

¼ teaspoon ground cumin

1 teaspoon salt, or more to taste

¼ cup (8 grams) chopped cilantro leaves

Combine all the ingredients except the cilantro in a high-speed blender and blend until smooth, adding more water if the soup is too thick. Add the cilantro and pulse until combined. Taste and adjust the seasonings with salt and lime juice if needed. Serve immediately, or cover and keep in the refrigerator until ready to serve.

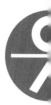

Entrées

Though we are taking a break from fiber during our juice-only programs, these programs (like all good things) must come to an end, or at least transition into the next good thing, which is eating! And eating fiber-filled greens, along with whole grains, nuts, and seeds in the LOVE*Lifestyle, is the way to go. Actually, unless you are on a juice-only cleanse, you'll be enjoying some of these very entrées! So eat, cleanse, and don't be deprived: You'll be enjoying a selection of generously filled wraps cleverly held together by a collard leaf, pesto and marinara noodles made from zucchini, a nut-based falafel that forgoes the fryer, and a raw lasagna to live for. Trust me, you'll be LOVE*ing every bite!

[239]

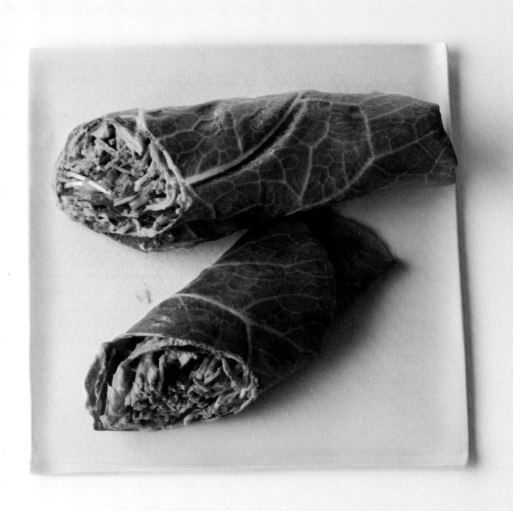

Lucky Lebanese Wraps

At Organic Avenue, collard greens are not just for salads and juicing. We also use them as a wrap in the raw, a convenient, chlorophyll-containing container for any number of fillings, this one Middle Eastern–inspired and based on tahini and sun-dried tomatoes.

The filling will keep for up to 5 days; store it (and the vegetable mixture) in the refrigerator and make a wrap at a time as you need them throughout the workweek.

Makes 4 wraps

Tahini Filling
(Makes about 1 cup/220 grams)

½ cup (120 grams) raw tahini
⅓ cup (15 grams) sun-dried tomatoes, soaked in water for 2 to 3 hours, drained, and chopped
2 garlic cloves, cut in half
¼ cup (60 milliliters) extra-virgin olive oil
½ cup (120 milliliters) water
1½ tablespoons fresh lemon juice
½ teaspoon salt
¼ teaspoon ground turmeric
¼ teaspoon ground cumin
Pinch of ground cayenne
½ teaspoon dried oregano

Wraps

2 medium carrots, cut into julienne
2 medium parsnips, cut into julienne
1 small celery root, cut into julienne
½ small red onion, thinly sliced
3 tablespoons extra-virgin olive oil
1 teaspoon dried sage
¼ teaspoon salt
¼ teaspoon freshly ground black pepper
4 large collard green leaves
4 tablespoons chopped fresh mint
4 handfuls of sunflower sprouts

[241]

Make the tahini filling: Combine all the ingredients in a food processor or blender and process until smooth.

Make the wraps: In a large bowl, combine the carrots, parsnips, celery root, red onion, oil, sage, salt, and pepper. Place a collard leaf bottom side up on a cutting board and using a sharp knife, shave off as much of the thick part of the stem as possible. Spread one quarter of the tahini filling over the leaf, leaving a ½-inch (1.25-centimeter) border on all sides. Add one quarter of the julienned vegetable mixture and sprinkle with 1 tablespoon of the mint and a handful of sunflower sprouts. Working from the end facing you, tightly roll the collard leaf away from you. Place seam side down, tuck in the sides, and cut the wrap in half using a serrated knife. Place on a plate; repeat with the remaining 3 wraps and filling. Serve immediately.

Variation: Happy Hummus Wrap

Substitute a scoop of Happy Hummus (page 225) for the tahini filling.

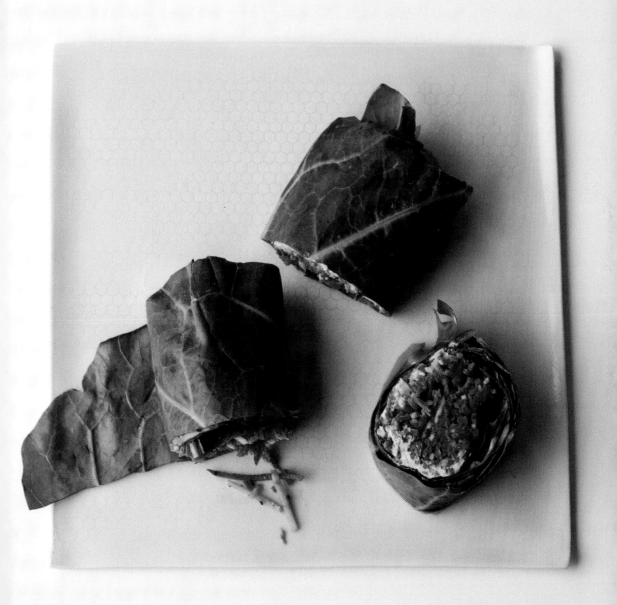

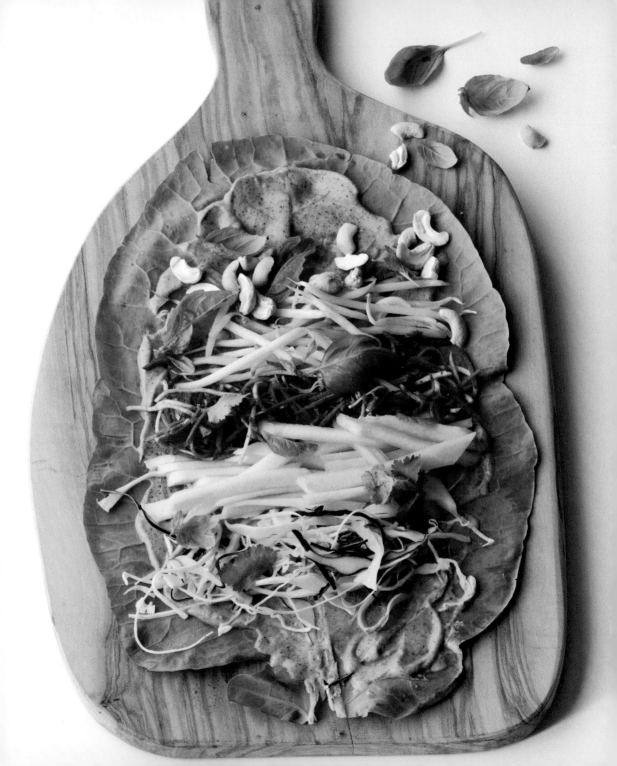

Thai Wrap with Thai Almond Cream and Sweet and Spicy Prune Dipping Sauce

This wrap, at once sweet, spicy, and tangy, is also a good protein source, thanks to the almond butter and cashews. Collard leaves do make a neat little wrapper—sturdy enough to support a substantial filling but tender enough to be enjoyed out of hand, a clever way of getting in your greens, and they are great for folks who are counting their carbs or calories.

The filling and dipping sauce will keep in the refrigerator for up to 5 days, so they can be made ahead and kept ready for rolling your wraps as you're ready for them.

Makes 4 wraps

Sweet and Spicy Prune Dipping Sauce

(Makes about ¾ cup/180 milliliters)

5 pitted prunes, soaked in water to cover for 2 to 3 hours and drained
2 tablespoons fresh lime juice
2 tablespoons coconut sugar
1½ teaspoons tamari
2 teaspoons sesame oil
½ cup (120 milliliters) water
Pinch of salt
4 pinches of red chile flakes

Thai Almond Cream

½ cup (4 ounces/110 grams) almond butter
2 tablespoons coconut sugar
1½ teaspoons fresh ginger juice
2 tablespoons fresh lime juice
1 tablespoon tamari
½ garlic clove, cut in half
2 tablespoons water

[245]

Wraps

4 large collard green leaves
1 cup (100 grams) shredded cabbage
1 mango, cut in half, pitted, peeled and flesh cut into long, thin strips
2 medium carrots, shredded
1 tablespoon chopped mint leaves
1 tablespoon chopped basil leaves
1 tablespoon chopped cilantro leaves
½ cup (50 grams) chopped cashews

Make the Sweet and Spicy Prune Dipping Sauce: Combine all the ingredients except the chile flakes in a blender and blend until smooth. Divide the sauce among 4 dipping bowls, add a pinch of chile flakes to each, and set aside.

Make the Thai Almond Cream: Rinse the blender, then combine all the ingredients in the blender and blend until smooth. Transfer to a bowl.

Assemble the wraps: Place a collard leaf bottom side up on a cutting board and using a sharp knife, shave off as much of the thick part of the stem as possible. Spread one quarter of the almond cream over the leaf, leaving a ½-inch (1.25-centimeter) border on all sides. Make a line of one quarter of the cabbage over the bottom third of the collard leaf; above the cabbage, make a line of one quarter of the mango; finish with a line of one quarter of the carrot. Sprinkle with one quarter of the mint, basil, and cilantro. Top with one quarter of the cashews. Working from the end facing you, tightly roll the collard leaf away from you. Place seam side down, tuck in the sides, and cut the wrap in half using a serrated knife. Place on a plate; repeat with the remaining 3 wraps and filling. Place a bowl of dipping sauce on each plate and serve.

Magic Mushroom Wrap with Creamy Kraut Filling

Our final wrap offering makes magic with mushrooms and spinach by treating them to a tangy, creamy, vegan variation on America's favorite, Thousand Island dressing, spiked with sauerkraut and finished with caraway. You'll find naturally fermented sauerkraut, full of live bacteria (the good guys!), in the refrigerated section of your natural food store; look for the words "raw" or "unpasteurized" on the label to be sure you get the benefits. The kraut filling doubles as a dip for crackers and crudités.

Makes 4 wraps

Creamy Kraut Filling
(Makes about 1½ cups/360 grams)

1 cup packed (200 grams) Confident Cashew Cream Cheese
  (page 216)
1 recipe Merry Marinara Sauce (page 261)
1 cup (170 grams) naturally fermented sauerkraut
1 tablespoon caraway seeds

Wraps
4 large collard green leaves
4 handfuls baby spinach leaves
1 recipe marinated mushrooms (page 262)

Make the Creamy Kraut Filling: In a medium bowl, combine all the ingredients.

Assemble the wraps: Place a collard leaf bottom side up on a cutting board and using a sharp knife, shave off as much of the thick part of the stem as possible. Spread one quarter of the kraut filling over the leaf, leaving a ½-inch (1.25-centimeter) border on all sides. Add a handful of spinach leaves and

[247]

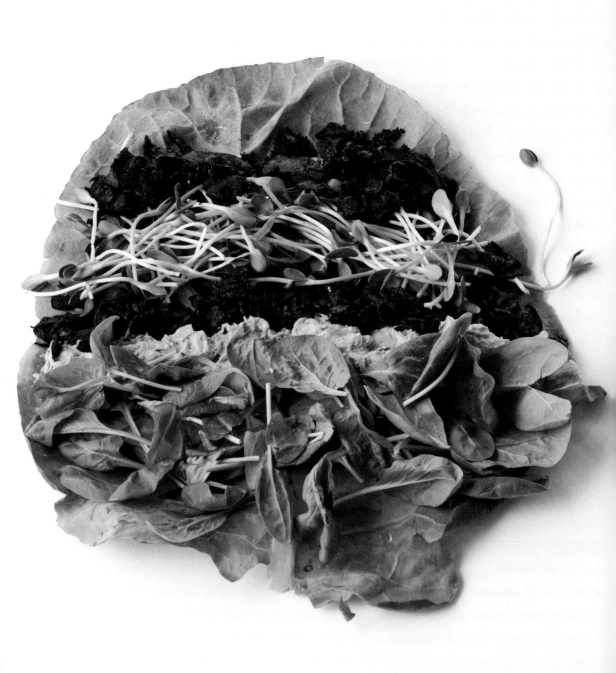

arrange one quarter of the marinated mushrooms on top. Working from the end facing you, tightly roll the collard leaf away from you. Place seam side down, tuck in the sides, and cut the wrap in half using a serrated knife. Place on a plate; repeat with the remaining 3 wraps and filling. Serve immediately.

SAVE YOUR SCRAPS

Don't let the trimmings from your collard green stems go to waste: save them, and when you pull out the juicer, run them through to include them in your next juice.

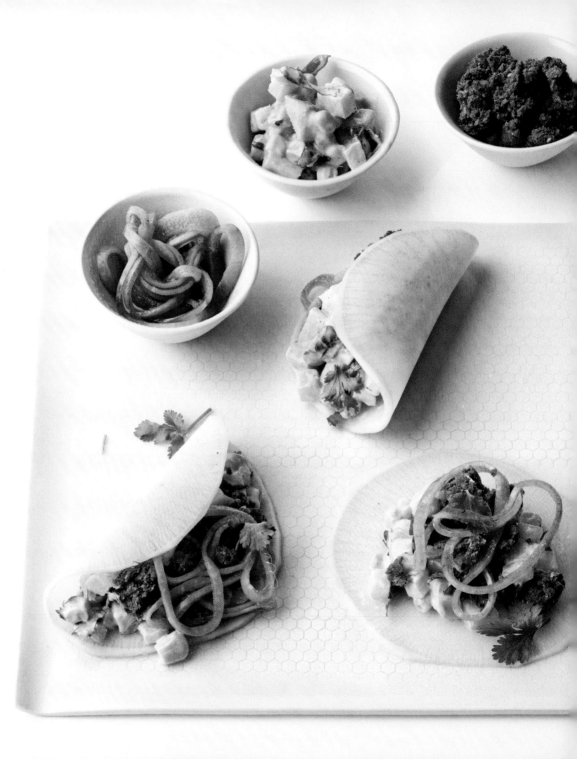

Tasty Taco with Chipotle Mango Corn Salsa and Pickled Red Onion

This Mexican-inspired three-part taco—including a sun-dried tomato–based filling, chipotle mango-corn salsa, and pickled red onion—makes for a slightly sweet and spicy meal with enough for leftovers. You'll have extra lime chipotle cream, some of which you can dollop on your tacos; save the rest to use another time as a sandwich spread or dip for crudités.

When you've finished your pickled red onions, don't discard the pickling liquid: Use it as the base of a salad dressing, or toss it with some shredded cabbage for a sweet and sour vegan coleslaw. Feel free to substitute any large root vegetable such as turnip or watermelon radish for the rutabaga taco "shell"; using a lettuce leaf as your taco wrapper is another fun option, and a time-saver to boot.

Makes 4 to 8 tacos, depending on the size of your wrapper and appetite

Pickled Onion

½ cup (120 milliliters) apple cider vinegar

[251]

½ cup (120 milliliters) water

½ teaspoon ground cinnamon

Pinch of ground cloves

1 medium red onion, sliced into thin rings

Lime-Chipotle Cream

(Makes about 1 cup/225 grams)

1½ cups (170 grams) cashews, soaked in water to cover overnight and drained

2 tablespoons fresh lime juice

¼ cup (60 milliliters) water

1 garlic clove, cut in half

½ teaspoon chipotle chile powder

½ teaspoon salt

Mango Corn Salsa

(Makes about 2 cups/300 grams)

1 mango, peeled, pitted, and cut into ¼-inch (6-millimeter) cubes
1½ cups (140 grams) fresh corn kernels
¼ cup (15 grams) chopped cilantro
⅓ cup Lime-Chipotle Cream (page 251)
1 tablespoon fresh lime juice
½ teaspoon salt

Taco Meat

(Makes about 2 cups/435 grams)

½ cup (60 grams) sunflower seeds, soaked in water to cover overnight and
    drained
¾ cup (30 grams) sun-dried tomatoes, soaked in water to cover for 2 to 3 hours
    and drained
1 small fresh plum tomato, chopped
1 small carrot, chopped
¼ yellow onion, roughly chopped
1 garlic clove
½ to 1 jalapeño chile, seeded
2 tablespoons chopped cilantro
3 tablespoons fresh lime juice
1 teaspoon chopped oregano leaves
½ teaspoon chipotle chile powder
¼ teaspoon ground cumin
¾ teaspoon salt
1 to 2 tablespoons water, as needed

1 rutabaga, thinly sliced and soaked in salted water for 1 hour
Cilantro leaves for garnish

[252]

Make the pickled onion: Combine the vinegar, water, cinnamon, and cloves in a medium bowl. Place the red onion slices in a glass jar, pour the vinegar mixture over them, cover, and refrigerate for at least 4 hours or overnight.

Make the Lime-Chipotle Cream: Combine all the ingredients in a food processor or high-speed blender and process until smooth.

Make the Mango Corn Salsa: Combine all the ingredients in a medium bowl.

Make the taco meat: In a food processor, combine all the ingredients and process until well combined and a little chunky; take care not to overprocess into a puree.

To assemble: Place a rutabaga slice on a plate and pat dry. Top with some taco meat and some Mango-Corn Salsa. Finish with a pickled onion ring and a dollop of Lime-Chipotle Cream if you like. Garnish with cilantro leaves. Repeat with the remaining rutabaga slices, filling, and toppings.

[253]

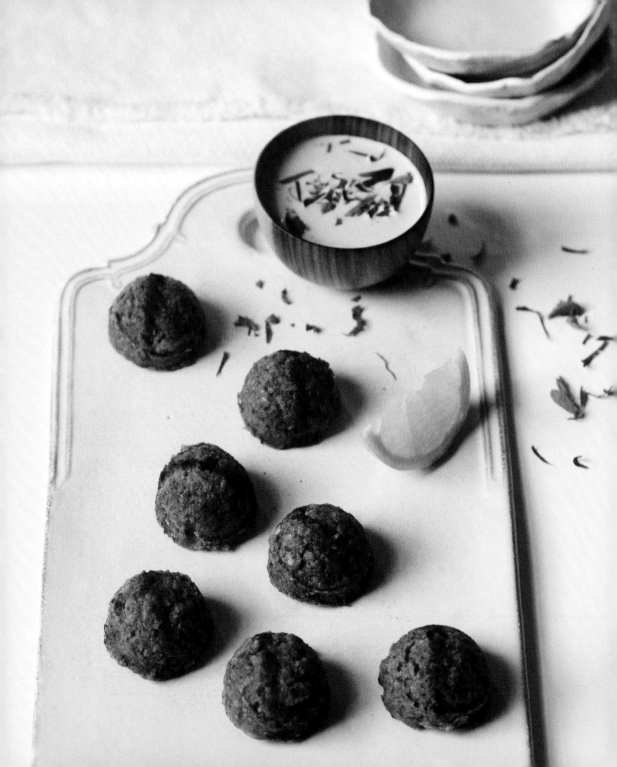

Fanciful Falafel with Lucky Lebanese Dip

Falafel without frying! Raw almonds in place of the traditional cooked chickpeas make Organic Avenue's version totally LOVE* friendly, while tasting remarkably like the classic recipe. It doubles easily; you could even triple or quadruple it, depending on the number of shelves in your dehydrator, for a great make-ahead party app. Or serve over a bed of shredded cabbage, salad style, which is how we do it at our Organic Avenue retail locations.

 If you don't have a 1-ounce cookie scoop, scoop 2 tablespoons of the mixture and form it into balls with your hands.

Makes about 30 pieces (serves 6)

1 cup (6 ounces/180 grams) raw almonds
2 tablespoons ground cumin
1 tablespoon onion powder
1 tablespoon ground coriander
½ teaspoon freshly ground black pepper
Pinch of ground cayenne
1½ teaspoons salt
½ cup packed (1 ounce/28 grams) parsley leaves
1 garlic clove, cut in half
1½ cups (8 ounces/225 grams) sunflower seeds, soaked in water to cover overnight
¼ cup (3 ounces/80 grams) tahini
Juice of 1 lemon
3 tablespoons (60 milliliters) extra-virgin olive oil
1 large scallion, light and green parts, minced
Paprika for dusting
2 cups (about 75 grams) shredded green or red cabbage, or a combination
Lucky Lebanese Dip (page 227)

Make the falafel: Put the almonds in a food processor and process to a powder; this will take about 2 minutes. Be careful not to overprocess or your almond powder will start to turn to almond butter. Transfer the almonds to a large bowl and add the cumin, onion powder, coriander, black pepper, cayenne, and salt.

[255]

Combine the parsley and garlic in the food processor (no need to rinse it first) and process until finely minced. Add the mixture to the almond powder mixture.

Drain the sunflower seeds and rinse them; drain again. Put them in the food processor (again, no need to rinse it), add 1 tablespoon water, and process to a coarse paste—you want it to remain a little chunky. Scrape the sides two or three times and add a little more water if needed. Transfer the sunflower paste to the almond powder mixture. Add the tahini, lemon juice, and oil and mix well with your hands, then mix in the scallions.

Using a 1-ounce cookie scoop, scoop the mixture onto two ParaFlexx-lined dehydrator sheets and sprinkle the falafel balls with paprika. Set the machine to 110°F (40°C) and dehydrate for 12 hours. Remove the falafel balls from the ParaFlexx and place them directly on the dehydrator's mesh screens. Dehydrate for another 5 hours, or until slightly crisp on the outside but moist on the inside.

Serve the falafel over the cabbage with the dip alongside.

FOOD COMBINING

First things first: I'd like you to be aware that a concept called food combining actually exists. It will be new to some of you; others may be familiar with it from Fit for Life, a health program from back in the eighties that popularized the concept. The idea behind food combining is that foods that take the same amount of time to digest combine easily together, and foods that take different lengths of time to digest can negatively affect digestion.

Enjoy a varied diet (emphasis on the enjoyment!) and consider the basic food combining guidelines that follow. But remember that they are guidelines and not set in stone, as when you're following the LOVE*Lifestyle you're already ahead of the game when it comes to digestion. But if you find your digestion is less than optimal or you're in a period of refining (see Top Five Food-Combining Tips, opposite), try following them more closely for some time and notice how you feel.

TOP FIVE FOOD-COMBINING TIPS

1. Combine greens freely: All greens go together well.
2. Eat fruit first thing in the morning, on its own, or take a break after a meal before eating your fruit for dessert. (Fruit digests very quickly and can interfere with the digestion of other foods.) Fruit and vegetable juice combinations are OK, as juicing requires little digestive work.
3. Eat melon on its own; it digests so quickly that it's best not to combine it with anything else, not even other fruits.
4. Combine proteins with vegetables.
5. Combine carbs with vegetables (you can't lose by partnering with a vegetable!).

TIP

When possible, avoid eating proteins and carbs at the same meal, as they digest at different rates. This isn't something we can always do in the real world, so you may want to think of it as a goal for a meal or two a day, or to follow more closely at times when you feel the need to fine-tune your digestion.

[257]

Plentiful Pesto Noodles

Pesto-standard pine nuts share the stage with walnuts in Organic Avenue's flavor-packed take on the classic. The key to packing your pesto with a punch is to be generous with your seasonings: lots of garlic and lemon, and don't skimp on the salt. Then do a final flavor check after tossing the pesto with your noodles just before serving.

The noodles, made from 100 percent zucchini, couldn't be simpler to make, once you've made a modest investment in a spiral slicer (see Food and Equipment Sources, page 317) or mandoline. The rule of thumb for making zucchini noodles is one zucchini per person, so if supper is for one or two, no need to "spiralize" all of your zucchini at once; just use as many zucchinis as you have diners and save the rest for another meal.

Serves 4 (makes about 1 cup/240 milliliters sauce)

Zucchini Noodles
4 medium zucchini, ends trimmed

Plentiful Pesto
5 garlic cloves, peeled
1 cup (3 ounces/90 grams) walnut halves
¼ cup (1 ounce/30 grams) pine nuts
½ teaspoon salt, or to taste
¼ teaspoon freshly ground black pepper
1 tablespoon fresh lemon juice, or to taste
2 cups (1 bunch/55 grams) packed basil leaves, plus a few leaves for garnish
⅔ cup (140 milliliters) extra-virgin olive oil

Plentiful Pine Nut Parmesan (page 223)

Make the Zucchini Noodles: Using a spiral slicer or mandoline, cut the zucchini into ribbon- or spaghetti-shape noodles and place them in a large bowl.

Make the Plentiful Pesto: In a food processor with the motor running, drop the garlic cloves through the hole in the top to mince. Add the walnuts, pine nuts, salt, and pepper and process until coarsely ground. Add the lemon juice and basil and process to mince the basil. With the motor running, drizzle in the oil through the hole in the top to incorporate.

To assemble: Add the pesto to the noodles and toss to coat. Divide among bowls, top with a little Parmesan, garnish with basil leaves, and serve.

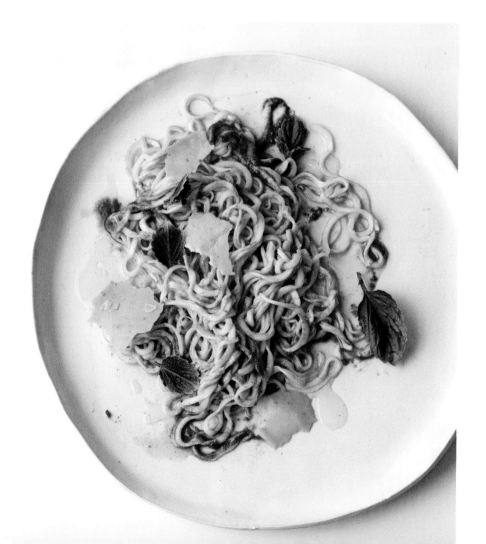

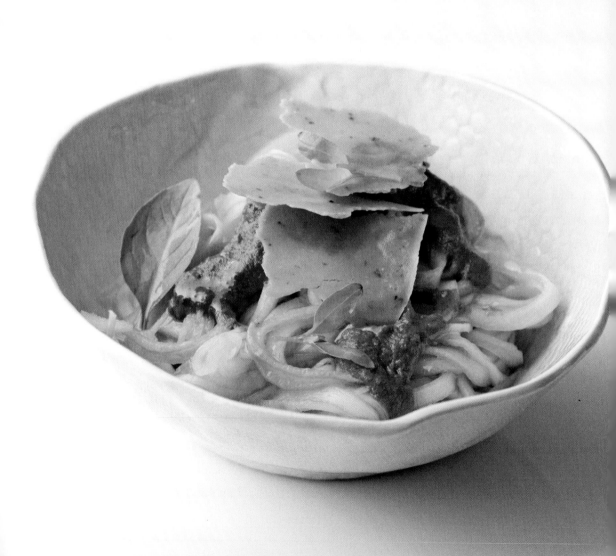

Merry Marinara Noodles

A combination of fresh and sun-dried tomatoes makes for a light and lively marinara with a distinctive depth. As I mentioned in the Plentiful Pesto Noodles recipe (page 258), the rule of thumb for making zucchini noodles is one zucchini per person, so go ahead and use as many zucchini as you have diners and save the rest for future meals.

Serves 6 (makes about 2 cups/480 milliliters sauce)

Zucchini Noodles
6 medium zucchini, ends trimmed

Merry Marinara Sauce
(Makes about 1 cup/240 milliliters)

2 plum tomatoes, roughly chopped
½ cup (20 grams) sun-dried tomatoes, soaked in water to cover for
   2 to 3 hours, drained, and chopped
½ cup (120 milliliters) extra-virgin olive oil
2 to 3 dates, soaked in water to cover for 2 to 3 hours, drained, and pitted
1 garlic clove, cut in half
4 teaspoons fresh lemon juice
1 teaspoon dried oregano

Plentiful Pine Nut Parmesan (page 223)
Basil leaves

[261]

Make the Zucchini Noodles: Using a spiral slicer or mandoline, cut the zucchini into ribbon- or spaghetti-shape noodles and place them in a large bowl.

Make the Merry Marinara Sauce: Combine all the ingredients in a food processor and pulse until well combined with some chunks remaining.

To assemble: Add the sauce to the noodles and toss to coat. Divide among bowls, top with a little Parmesan, garnish with basil leaves, and serve.

Pleasing Pasta with Truffle Cream Sauce

Truffle oil and an option for a sprinkling of shaved truffle take this healthful pasta and veggie dish into the realm of luxury and extreme deliciousness. If you're looking for a way to get more sea vegetables into your life, the raw kelp noodle option is a good place to start. That's because these clear noodles, loaded with all-important iodine and other trace minerals, have no seaweed taste! Plus they have almost zero calories and carbs, nice for those of us watching ourselves in those departments. If, on the other hand, you're looking for some serious cooked vegan comfort food, then the mung bean noodles are the way to go. Kelp noodles can be found in some natural food stores or online (see Food and Equipment Sources, page 317) and mung bean noodles can be found in some natural food stores and Asian groceries. Truffle oil can be found in some groceries and specialty foods stores.

You'll have some marinated mushrooms left over, which you can add to a salad such as the Mighty Mushroom and Fennel Salad on page 205.

Serves 4

Marinated Mushrooms

(Makes about 3 cups/200 grams)

½ pound (220 grams) portobello mushrooms
½ pound (220 grams) cremini mushrooms
⅓ cup (70 milliliters) extra-virgin olive oil
¼ teaspoon dried thyme
½ teaspoon onion powder
¼ teaspoon salt
Pinch of freshly ground black pepper

Creamy Cashew Sauce

Makes about 1½ cups/350 milliliters

1½ cups (6 ounces/170 grams) cashews, soaked in water to cover overnight and drained

1 tablespoon white chickpea miso

1 teaspoon onion powder

2 teaspoons fresh lemon juice, or more to taste

½ teaspoon garlic powder

1 teaspoon grated lemon zest

1 garlic clove, cut in half

½ cup (120 milliliters) water

2 teaspoons extra-virgin olive oil

½ teaspoon truffle oil

¾ teaspoon salt, or more to taste

¼ teaspoon freshly ground black pepper

One 12-ounce (340-gram) package kelp noodles; one 7-ounce (200-gram) package mung bean fettuccine, cooked; or three 2-ounce (56-gram) packages mung bean thread noodles, cooked

[263]

2 large kale leaves, finely chopped or shredded in a food processor

1 red bell pepper, cored, seeded, and cut into strips

2 tablespoons finely chopped dill

Fresh truffle shavings (optional)

Make the Marinated Mushrooms: Remove the gills from the underside of the por-tobello mushroom stems by scraping them off with a spoon. Thinly slice both the portobello and cremini mushrooms, place them in a bowl, and toss with the oil to coat. Add the remaining ingredients and toss to coat. Spread the mush-rooms evenly onto ParaFlexx-lined dehydrator sheets. Set the machine to 110°F (40°C) and dehydrate for 4 to 5 hours, turning them a few times and keeping them more or less bunched together to retain their moisture, until moist and juicy and slightly crisp on the outside.

Make the Creamy Cashew Sauce: Combine all the ingredients in a blender and blend on high speed until smooth.

To assemble: Place the noodles in a large bowl and toss with enough sauce to coat (there may be some left over). Add as many of the marinated mushrooms as you like, the kale, bell pepper strips, and dill and toss to combine. Taste and add more salt or lemon juice if needed. Top with the truffle shavings, if using.

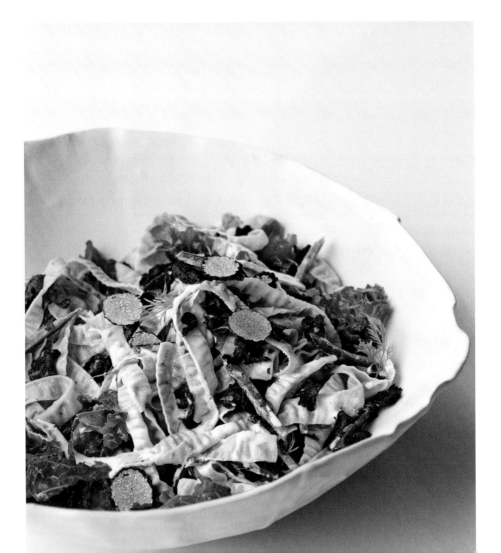

Live Lasagna

Our lasagna, made from thinly sliced raw zucchini rather than cooked wheat pasta, along with a host of living sauces, pesto, and cheese, is an elegant dish, something to dress up for and serve with your finest silverware. If you've got a mandoline, this is a good time to pull it out and turn it to the finest setting for light-as-a-feather lasagna noodles that will soak in the sauces.

While our recipe involves making several different fillings, it can be simplified in any number of ways: Skip the pesto or one of the sauces, skip the cheese, or use just the tomato sauce (scaling up the amount), depending on what you have on hand and what you have time for. Any leftover pesto, sauces, or cheese can be used for dipping or serving with zucchini noodles (page 258) or for making additional servings of Live Lasagna.

Serves 6 to 8

Walnut Bolognese Sauce

(Makes about 1½ cups/250 grams)

[265]

1½ cups (150 grams) walnuts, soaked in water to cover overnight and drained
¼ cup (10 grams) sun-dried tomatoes, soaked in water for 2 to 3 hours, drained, and chopped
1 date, soaked in water to cover for 2 to 3 hours, drained, pitted, and roughly chopped
1 tablespoon extra-virgin olive oil
1 tablespoon white chickpea miso
½ teaspoon dried oregano
½ teaspoon dried sage
Pinch of ground cayenne
Salt if needed

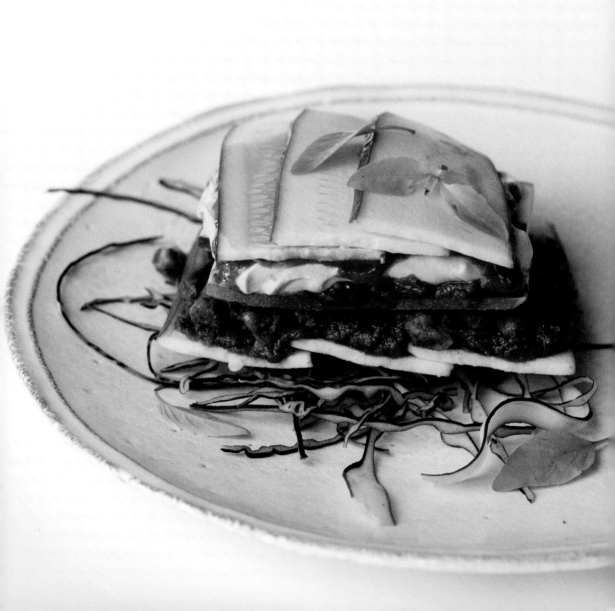

Cheese Sauce

(Makes about 1½ cups/300 grams)

1 cup (130 grams) macadamia nuts
½ cup (65 grams) pine nuts
½ yellow bell pepper, cored, seeded, and roughly chopped
2 tablespoons water, or more if needed
1 tablespoon fresh lemon juice, or more to taste
¼ teaspoon dried thyme
¼ teaspoon ground turmeric
¼ teaspoon salt, or more to taste

½ small red cabbage, cored and shredded
2 to 4 medium zucchini, ends trimmed, sliced horizontally on the finest setting
  of a mandoline or very thinly sliced
Merry Marinara Sauce (page 261)
Plentiful Pesto (page 258)

Make the Walnut Bolognese Sauce: Combine all the ingredients in a food processor and pulse until well combined with some chunks remaining; do not process until smooth. Taste and season with salt if needed.

[267]

Make the Cheese Sauce: Combine all the ingredients in a blender and blend on high speed until smooth, adding more water if the sauce is too thick. Taste and adjust the seasonings with salt and lemon juice if needed.

Assemble the lasagna: Arrange a handful of cabbage on a dinner plate. Top with 3 zucchini slices, placed side by side horizontally. Spread a little marinara sauce on top, then spread some Bolognese over the marinara sauce. Top with 3 more zucchini slices, placed vertically this time. Top with some more marinara sauce and Bolognese sauce, followed by some cheese sauce and pesto. End with a final 3 horizontal zucchini slices. Top with a few basil leaves. Repeat with the remaining zucchini, sauces, cheese, and pesto. (Note: These are suggestions; feel free to layer in whatever order with whatever sauces you like!)

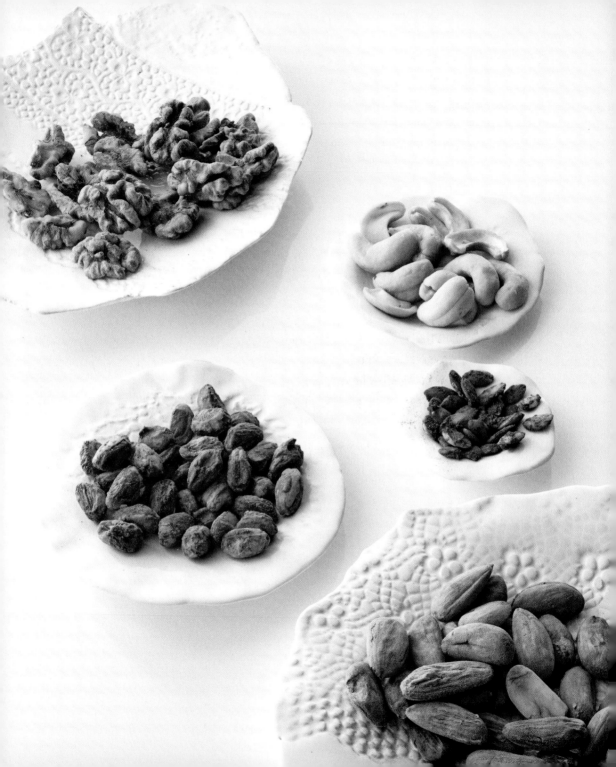

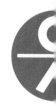

Nut and Seed Snacks

Our little friends in the nut and seed family are perfectly portable snack items, either eaten by the handful raw or treated to some salt, sugar, spice, and other nice things and crisped up in the dehydrator, the food of LOVE* answer to roasting nuts and seeds while keeping them raw.

Nuts and seeds are a go-to LOVE*Food, as they are full of protein, fiber, B vitamins, and a host of minerals; they'll fill you up and keep you going while cycling or hiking, post-workout, or as a between-meals tide-me-over. Once you have the method down—soaking nuts in salt water overnight, then tossing with spices and dehydrating them—feel free to mix and match spices: Salty, sweet, spicy, tangy, or all of the above are excellent ways to flavor your nuts and seeds. Bag a few and you're out the door ready to face the day with LOVE*.

[269]

Adorable Almonds

The almond is a favorite on-the-go energy food. And almonds consistently top the charts in nutrition: They are good for the brain and heart, they help regulate cholesterol, and they have a limited effect on blood sugar. The simple dehydrator technique for "roasting" almonds crisps them up while keeping them raw.

Makes 1 pound (450 grams)

1 pound (450 grams) raw almonds
2 teaspoons salt

Put the almonds in a large bowl and add water to cover. Stir in 1 teaspoon of the salt, cover with a kitchen towel, and leave to soak overnight. Drain, rinse, and return the almonds to the bowl. Add the remaining 1 teaspoon salt and stir well to coat.

Arrange the almonds on ParaFlexx-lined dehydrator sheets in one layer. Turn the machine to 110°F (40°C) and dehydrate for about 24 hours, until completely dry and crisp. Store in an airtight container.

Capable Cashews

Is it possible that consuming cashews regularly could protect or improve your eyesight? Because of their high amounts of zeaxanthin, a carotenoid that acts as an antioxidant in the eyes, cashews may increase the health of your eyes and prevent macular degeneration as we age. Let's get started now!

Makes 1 pound (450 grams)

1 pound (450 grams) cashews
2 teaspoons salt

Put the cashews in a large bowl and add water to cover. Stir in 1 teaspoon of the salt, cover with a kitchen towel, and leave to soak overnight. Drain, rinse, and return the cashews to the bowl. Add the remaining 1 teaspoon salt and stir well to coat.

Arrange the cashews on ParaFlexx-lined dehydrator sheets in one layer. Turn the machine to 110°F (40°C) and dehydrate for about 24 hours, until completely dry and crisp. Store in an airtight container.

[271]

Memorable Moroccan Cashews

Not only do cashews have a lower fat content than most other nuts, but approximately 75 percent of their fat is unsaturated fatty acid, a heart-healthy monounsaturated fat. Add to that good amounts of B vitamins, magnesium and a host of other minerals, and plenty of protein and fiber and you can't go wrong with a handful of cashews when you're hungry—especially with the array of herbs and spices you'll enjoy with every bite of these!

Makes 1 pound (450 grams)

1 pound (450 grams) cashews
2¼ teaspoons salt
1 cup (30 grams) chopped parsley
1 cup (30 grams) chopped cilantro
2 tablespoons fresh lemon juice
1 garlic clove, cut in half
1½ tablespoons ground cumin
1½ tablespoons paprika
1 teaspoon ground cardamom
¼ teaspoon ground cayenne

Put the cashews in a large bowl and add water to cover. Stir in 1 teaspoon of the salt, cover with a kitchen towel, and leave to soak overnight. Drain, rinse, and return the cashews to the bowl.

Combine the remaining 1¼ teaspoons salt, the parsley, cilantro, lemon juice, garlic, cumin, paprika, cardamom, and cayenne in a food processor and process until smooth. Add the mixture to the nuts and stir well to coat.

Arrange the cashews on ParaFlexx-lined dehydrator sheets in one layer. Turn the machine to 110°F (40°C) and dehydrate for about 24 hours, until completely dry and crisp. Store in an airtight container.

Perfectly Peppered Walnuts

Sometimes salt and pepper is all that's needed to satisfy, as in this simple brain-healthy walnut nibble. Walnuts are high in antioxidants and omega-3 fatty acids to keep you at your best throughout the day and also to reach and maintain long-term health goals. So pop some peppered walnuts often and you're sure to stay at the top of your game!

Makes 1 pound (450 grams)

1 pound (450 grams) walnuts
2 teaspoons salt
2 teaspoons freshly ground black pepper

Put the walnuts in a large bowl and add water to cover. Stir in 1 teaspoon of the salt, cover with a kitchen towel, and leave to soak overnight. Drain, rinse, and return the walnuts to the bowl. Add the remaining 1 teaspoon salt and the pepper and stir well to coat.

    Arrange the walnuts on ParaFlexx-lined dehydrator sheets in one layer. Turn the machine to 110°F (40°C) and dehydrate for about 24 hours, until completely dry and crisp. Store in an airtight container.

[273]

Chipper Chipotle Pistachios

This little green nut is a favorite of many, and full of many of my favorite nutrients, including vitamin B_6, vitamin E, copper, manganese, calcium, iron, magnesium, zinc, and selenium. We spice ours with chipotle chile powder, made from ground dried smoked jalapeños, and finish with an accent of lemon. Chipotle chile powder can be found in some supermarkets and Mexican groceries.

Makes 1 pound (450 grams)

1 pound (450 grams) shelled pistachios
2 teaspoons salt
1 teaspoon chipotle chile powder
5 tablespoons fresh lemon juice

Put the pistachios in a large bowl and add water to cover. Stir in 1 teaspoon of the salt, cover with a kitchen towel, and leave to soak overnight. Drain, rinse, and return the pistachios to the bowl. Add the remaining 1 teaspoon salt, the chipotle powder, and lemon juice and stir well to coat.

[274]

Arrange the pistachios on ParaFlexx-lined dehydrator sheets in one layer. Turn the machine to 110°F (40°C) and dehydrate for about 24 hours, until completely dry and crisp. Store in an airtight container.

Spicy Pumpkin Seeds

Known as *pepitas* in Mexico, where they are a common ingredient, here this little seed gets treated to a mixture of Mexican flavorings including chipotle chile, cumin, and lime juice. While you're enjoying them, your hair, nails, skin, eyes, and overall immune system will be getting a fair amount of support from their zinc content; the World Health Organization recommends eating pumpkin seeds as a good way of taking in this nutrient.

1 pound (450 grams) hulled pumpkin seeds (*pepitas*; not roasted)
2 teaspoons salt
1½ tablespoons paprika
1 tablespoon ground cumin
2 teaspoons chipotle chile powder
Pinch of ground cayenne
3 tablespoons fresh lime juice

Put the pumpkin seeds in a large bowl and add water to cover. Stir in 1 teaspoon of the salt, cover with a kitchen towel, and leave to soak overnight. Drain, rinse, and return the pumpkin seeds to the bowl. Add the remaining 1 teaspoon salt, the paprika, cumin, chipotle powder, cayenne, and lime juice and stir well to coat.

Arrange the pumpkin seeds on ParaFlexx-lined dehydrator sheets in one layer. Turn the machine to 110°F (40°C) and dehydrate for about 24 hours, until completely dry and crisp. Store in an airtight container.

Nice Nut Crunch

These nuts are sweet, slightly salty, and smoky from the mesquite powder (see Food and Equipment Sources, page 317), and you'll be breaking out packets of them on the trail, in the office, or first thing in the morning—just about any time is a good time!

Makes 1 pound (450 grams)

8 ounces (225 grams) almonds
¼ teaspoon plus a pinch of salt
8 ounces (225 grams) cashews
½ cup (60 grams) coconut sugar
3 tablespoons cocoa powder
2 teaspoons vanilla powder (see Note, page 162)
1 teaspoon mesquite powder
1 tablespoon cacao nibs
1 tablespoon coconut oil

Put the almonds in a large bowl and add water to cover (leave the cashews dry). Add the pinch of salt, cover with a kitchen towel, and leave to soak overnight. Drain, rinse, and return the almonds to the bowl. Add the cashews, the remaining ¼ teaspoon salt, the coconut sugar, cocoa powder, vanilla powder, mesquite powder, and cacao nibs and stir well to coat.

Spread the mixture over a ParaFlexx-lined dehydrator sheet in one layer. Turn the machine to 110°F (40°C) and dehydrate for about 24 hours, until completely dry and crisp. Remove from the dehydrator and break into large pieces. Place in a large bowl, add the coconut oil, and mix it in well. Let the coconut oil dry on the nuts and firm up (placing it in the refrigerator will speed up the process), then break into bite-size pieces. Store in an airtight container.

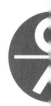

Sweet Treats

These are the treats that vegan dreams are made of, and their seductive sweetness keeps everyone, regardless of food persuasion, coming back for seconds. Using luxurious and sometimes unexpected ingredients such as young coconut, raw cocoa power, avocado, and coconut sugar, a new realm of unprocessed dessert goodness is born: You're going to LOVE* it! And there are surprises: Who would have known you could culture coconut into yogurt, make tapioca from chia seeds, or turn avocado into mousse? Granola, too, does a double take, sweetened with orange juice and dates, with buckwheat rather than oats providing its backbone. Read on for more of this dessert magic!

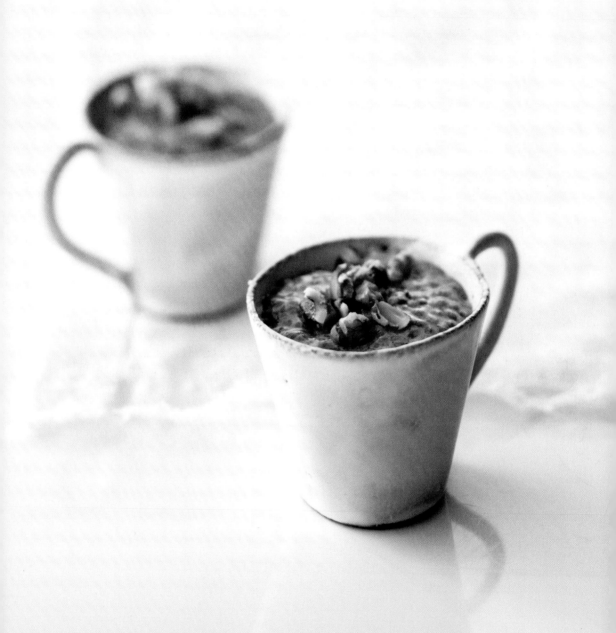

Cherished Chia Tapioca

This is a little different from the tapioca pudding many of us grew up on, with totally vegan ingredients and superfood chia seeds standing in for the tapioca pearls. Chia seeds are an excellent source of calcium, iron, protein, fiber, omega-3 fatty acids, and other nutrients. And the fun part is that when you add liquid to them, they swell up and thicken—no simmering required—to "cook up" this pudding while keeping it totally raw.

Serves 4

¼ cup (35 grams) Brazil nuts
2 cups (470 milliliters) water
⅓ cup (35 grams) coconut sugar
½ cup (40 grams) chia seeds
2 teaspoons vanilla powder (see Note, page 162)
Pinch of salt

Combine the Brazil nuts and water and leave to soak overnight (soak them right in a blender to save on time and cleaning). The next day, blend until smooth. Strain through a nut milk bag or a strainer lined with cheesecloth into a bowl.

Whisk together the coconut sugar, chia seeds, vanilla powder, and salt in a separate bowl. Add the Brazil nut milk and whisk until the dry ingredients are completely incorporated. Cover and refrigerate for at least 3 hours for the chia seeds to swell and thicken the liquid. Serve cold.

[279]

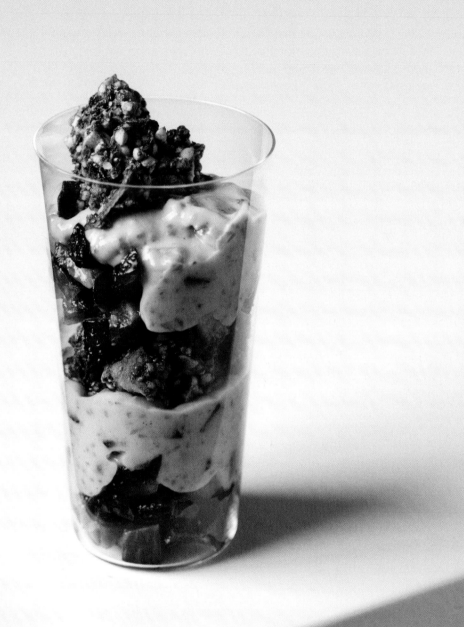

Soulful Strawberry Chia Custard

Red on white makes a striking presentation for this sweet treat, and fiber-rich chia seeds, with their thickening powers, niftily turn the yogurt into custard. The jam is delicious solo as well—spooned onto crackers and licked from fingers are two nice ways to go! Or forgo the jam and stick with the yogurt, fresh strawberries, and chia for simplicity's sake.

Serves 4 to 6

Strawberry Jam

2 cups (220 grams) strawberries, hulled and cut in half
1 cup (150 grams) dates, soaked in water to cover for 2 to 3 hours, drained, and pitted
½ cup (120 milliliters) water

Custard

1½ cups (360 grams) Cool Coconut Yogurt (page 283)
1 cup (130 grams) hulled and minced strawberries
⅓ cup (60 grams) chia seeds

[281]

Make the strawberry jam: Combine the strawberries, dates, and water in a blender and blend until smooth, scraping down the sides of the machine once or twice as needed.

Make the custard: Combine the yogurt, strawberries, and strawberry jam. Whisk in the chia seeds, cover, and refrigerate for at least 3 hours for the chia seeds to swell and thicken the liquid. Serve cold.

> **Intelligence precedes the body. The mind gets there first, and the body may take a while. Be patient, and be generous with the LOVE*."**
>
> **—DENISE MARI**

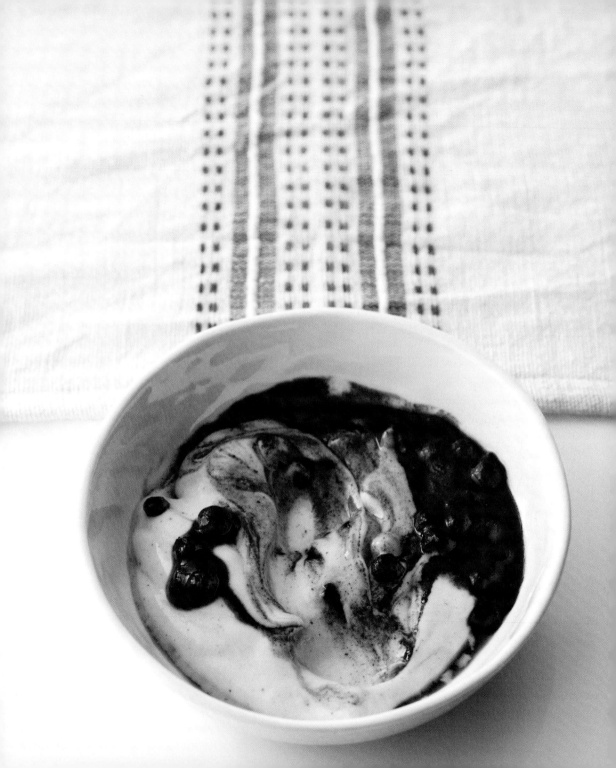

Cool Coconut Yogurt

Slightly sweet, totally satisfying, and packed with healthy fats to fuel you through the morning, this coconut-based yogurt is a breakfast for champions, even more so if you top it with Gracious Granola (page 285). Dairy-free acidophilus powder, which can be found in the refrigerated area of your natural food store's supplement section, works to ferment the coconut meat, transforming it into a totally vegan yogurt full of gut-healthy probiotic goodness.

You decide whether to include sweetener depending on your taste and how you plan to serve your yogurt, be it as an after-dinner treat or first thing in the morning for breakfast; here we use light-colored coconut blossom sugar (see Food and Equipment Sources, page 317) as our sweetener to maintain the coconut's creamy white color, but if it's not available, feel free to substitute regular powdered coconut sugar or the vegan sweetener of your choice.

Makes about 6 cups (1.5 liters)

2 pounds (1 kilogram) fresh coconut meat
1½ cups (350 milliliters) fresh coconut water
½ teaspoon dairy-free acidophilus powder
½ cup (100 grams) coconut blossom sugar (optional)
1 teaspoon vanilla powder (see Note, page 162)

[283]

Combine the coconut meat, coconut water, acidophilus, and coconut blossom sugar, if using, in a high-speed blender and blend until silky smooth, adding more coconut water if needed and scraping the sides of the machine as needed. This will take up to 5 minutes.

Put the mixture in a nonreactive bowl or container and leave it in a warm place for 12 hours to ferment.

Stir in the vanilla powder, pour the yogurt into containers, and refrigerate until ready to serve.

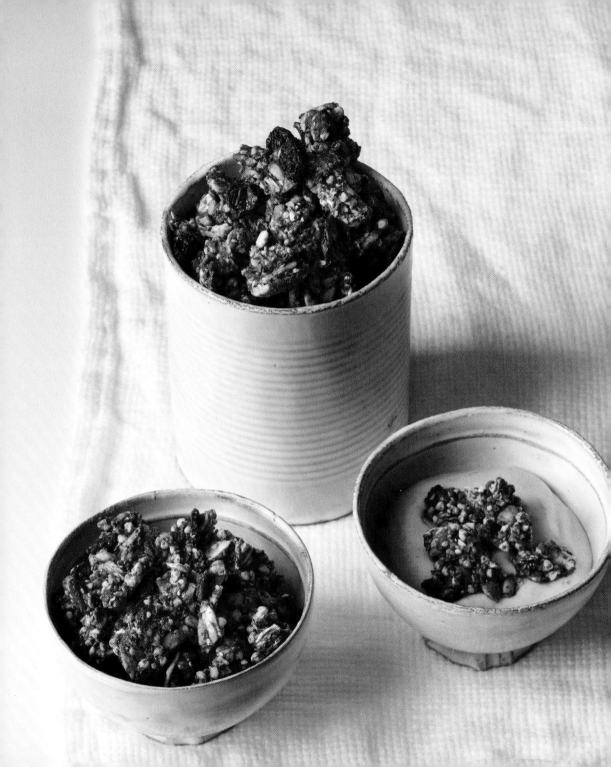

Gracious Granola

Organic Avenue's granola is not only gluten-free; it's oat-free and nut-free as well. In place of the standard base of ingredients, we use buckwheat, which when soaked and dehydrated gives our granola a delightfully light crunch. Then we add an assortment of superfoods including hemp seeds, chia seeds, and goji berries to take it up a few more notches. Mesquite powder, a superfood favored by native peoples of South and North America, adds an element of malty sweetness; increase the amount to further the effect. It's available at some natural food stores and online (see Food and Equipment Sources, page 317).

Don't be daunted by the long ingredient list; feel free to double up on some of the seeds and omit others, and if you don't have goji berries on hand, you can double the raisins or substitute another dried fruit. Eat out of hand for a between-meal tide-me-over sweet, sprinkle over Cool Coconut Yogurt (page 283), or pour some Appealing Almond Mylk or Creative Cashew Mylk (page 185 or 187) over a bowlful.

Makes 2 dehydrator sheets full (about 8 cups granola)

1 cup (225 grams) untoasted buckwheat groats   [285]
½ cup (70 grams) pumpkin seeds
½ cup (70 grams) sunflower seeds
¾ cup (110 grams) dates, pitted
¾ cup (175 ml) Outstanding Orange Juice (page 139)
Zest of 1 orange
1 cup (60 grams) unsweetened coconut flakes
½ cup (60 grams) hemp seeds
½ cup (80 grams) chia seeds
½ cup (60 grams) goji berries
½ cup (60 grams) raisins
¼ cup (30 grams) coconut sugar
½ cup (60 grams) maple sugar (or substitute another ¼ cup coconut sugar to
   keep it raw)
¼ cup (35 grams) lucuma powder
2 tablespoons cacao nibs

2 tablespoons mesquite powder

1 tablespoon vanilla powder (see Note, page 162)

1½ teaspoons ground cinnamon

¼ teaspoon salt

In a large bowl, combine the buckwheat, pumpkin seeds, and sunflower seeds; add water to cover by a few inches, cover with a dish towel, and soak overnight.

In a container with a lid, combine the dates, orange juice, and orange zest; cover and place in the refrigerator to soak for at least 3 hours or overnight.

Drain the soaked buckwheat, pumpkin seeds, and sunflower seeds. Rinse and drain again. Return the buckwheat and seeds to the bowl.

Put the soaked dates with the orange juice in a food processor and process until smooth. Transfer to the bowl with the buckwheat and seeds.

In a separate bowl, combine the coconut flakes, hemp seeds, chia seeds, goji berries, raisins, coconut sugar, maple sugar, lucuma powder, cacao nibs, mesquite powder, vanilla powder, cinnamon, and salt and stir to combine. Add the mixture to the buckwheat mixture and stir well to distribute the ingredients evenly.

Divide the mixture between two ParaFlexx-lined dehydrator sheets about ½ inch (1.25 centimeters) thick. Turn the machine to 110ºF (40ºC) and dehydrate for about 12 hours. Break the granola into pieces and dehydrate for 2 to 3 more hours, to desired crunchiness (just make sure it is completely dried to ensure the longest shelf life). It will crisp up a little more as it cools. The granola will keep for 2 months or more in an airtight container.

CEREAL OR BARS: YOU CHOOSE

If your breakfast is more of a grab-and-go than a sit-down-with-a-spoon, you might want to make granola bars: After dehydrating your granola for 12 hours, rather than breaking the granola into pieces, flip the whole sheet onto a mesh dehydrator screen and dehydrate for another 2 to 3 hours, then break into large bar-size pieces. Store in an airtight container, or individually wrap the bars for convenience.

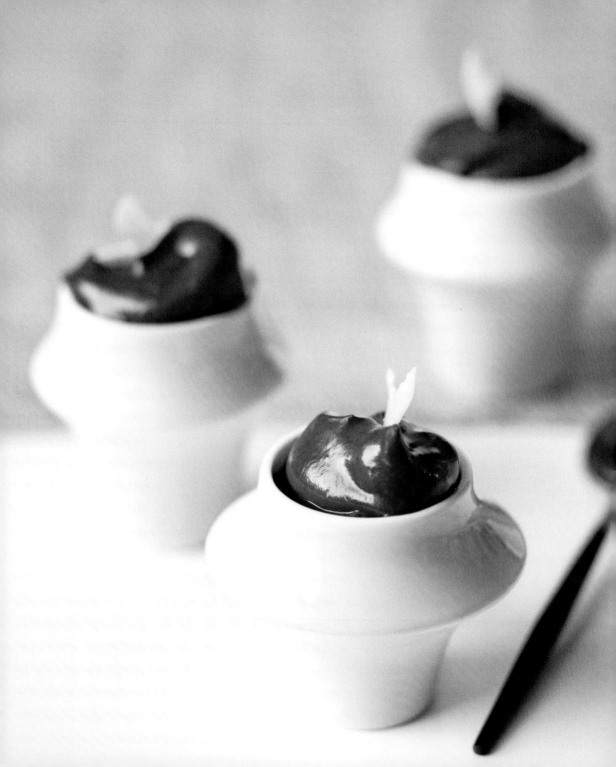

Magnificent Chocolate Mousse

Did you know that the avocado is a fruit, not a vegetable? A fruit of distinction, we might add, for it contains more fiber than any other fruit (add that to the list of avocado's heart-protective qualities!), and while we use this fruit in savory soups and guac, its creamy nature and mild flavor also mean it can double as a dessert base in many raw recipes, such as this deep chocolate vegan mousse spiked with a generous amount of espresso (consider using decaf if you're serving it after dinner).

Serves 8

1½ cups (360 milliliters) water
2 tablespoons fine instant espresso powder
5 ripe avocados, pitted and peeled
½ cup (1½ ounces/40 grams) cocoa powder
1 cup (4 ounces/120 grams) coconut sugar
½ cup (2 ounces/60 grams) maple sugar (or substitute another ½ cup coconut
   sugar to keep your mousse raw)
2 teaspoons vanilla powder (see Note, page 162)   [289]
¼ teaspoon salt

Warm the water in a small bowl or mug; whisk in the espresso powder to dissolve it. Combine the remaining ingredients in a food processor or high-speed blender, add the dissolved espresso, and process for about 2 minutes, scraping the sides once or twice, until silky smooth. Transfer to a container, cover, and refrigerate for a couple of hours to firm up, then spoon into dessert bowls and serve.

Variation: Cinnamon Chocolate Mousse

Replace the espresso powder with ¼ teaspoon ground cinnamon (in which case you don't need to heat the water).

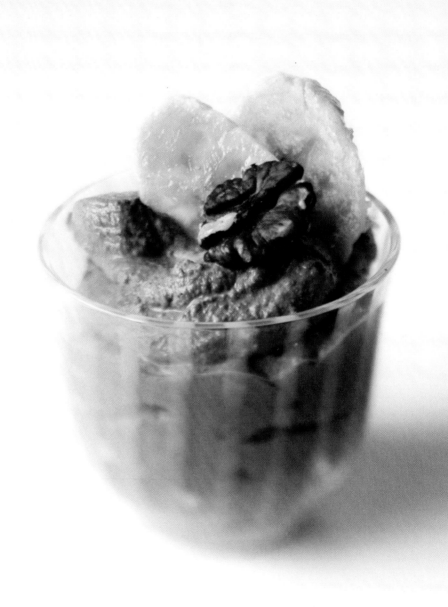

Wonderful Walnut Banana Pudding

Bananas serve as a base and give body to many of our smoothies; similarly they can work their magic in puddings to thicken and bind while simultaneously sweetening them. Antioxidant-rich walnuts add to the experience; make sure you buy yours from a store with good turnover, as walnuts tend to go rancid quickly, and store them in the refrigerator.

Serves 4 to 6

1½ cups (150 grams) walnuts, soaked in water to cover overnight and drained
1 ripe banana, broken into pieces
½ cup (120 milliliters) water
¾ cup (90 grams) coconut sugar
1 tablespoon fresh lemon juice
½ teaspoon vanilla powder (see Note, page 162)
½ teaspoon ground cinnamon
¼ teaspoon salt

In a blender, combine all the ingredients and blend from low to high speed [291] until silky smooth, stopping to scrape the sides of the machine once or twice. Transfer to a container, cover, and refrigerate for a couple of hours to firm up, then spoon into dessert bowls and serve.

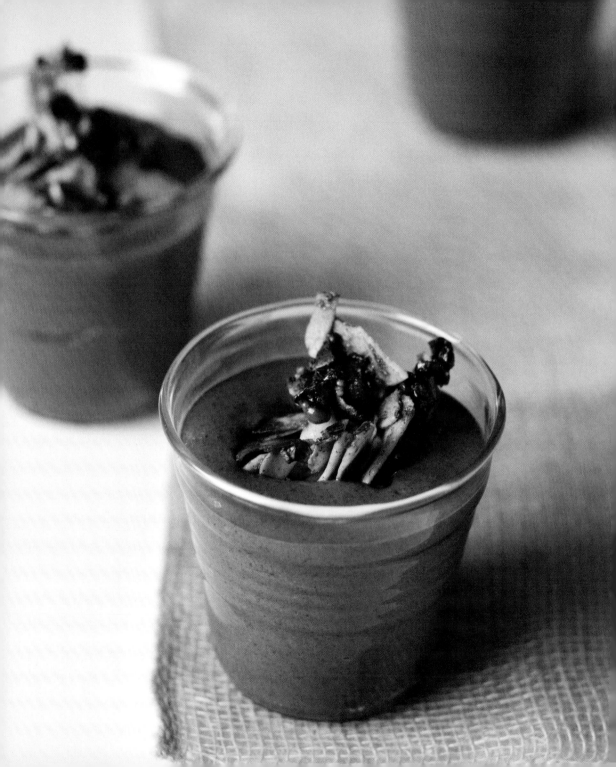

Heavenly Cardamom Chocolate Hemp Pudding

Hemp seeds, the source of the hemp we're using in this dessert, contain no psychedelic properties; what they do contain is a very absorbable form of amino acids that helps rebuild muscle. In fact, hemp protein contains all twenty-one known amino acids and all nine essential amino acids, making it a near complete vegan protein source—and a fully complete source of deliciousness when it's blended with chocolate into this silky smooth, touch-of-heaven hemp seed pudding.

Serves 4 to 6

1¾ cups (240 grams) hemp seeds
1 cup (120 grams) coconut sugar
1 cup (240 milliliters) Clearly Coconut Water (page 145) or bottled raw coconut water
½ cup (40 grams) cocoa powder
2 tablespoons cacao nibs
1 teaspoon fresh lemon juice
½ teaspoon ground cardamom
Pinch of salt

[293]

In a blender, combine all the ingredients and blend from low to high speed until silky smooth, stopping to scrape the sides of the machine once or twice. Transfer to a container, cover, and refrigerate for a couple of hours to firm up, then spoon into dessert bowls and serve.

DID YOU KNOW?
Hemp seeds have an excellent omega-6 to omega-3 fatty acid ratio, making them a top source of essential fatty acids.

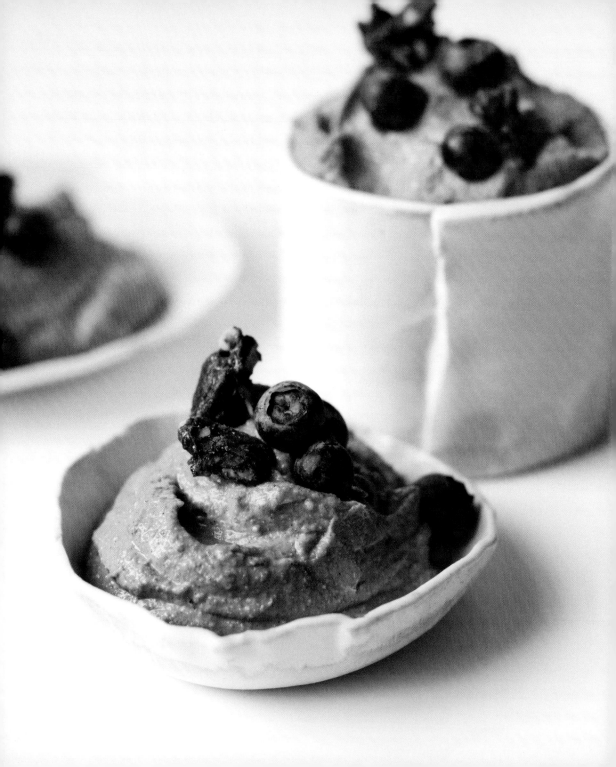

Peaceful Pecan Pie Pudding

Traditional pecan pie takes hours to make and is filled with corn syrup, white flour, and butter; this pie-pudding can be made in five minutes and is totally vegan, but it still boasts that unmistakable pecan pie flavor. The sweetener responsible for that flavor is maple sugar, made from the dried sap of the maple tree. While maple sugar is not a raw food, it is full of health-supportive minerals, including potassium, calcium, magnesium, manganese, zinc, and phosphorus, and favoring it is a good way of supporting the maple growers of North America and in doing so staying close to the local foods movement.

Serves 4 to 6

1½ cups (210 grams) pecans, soaked in water to cover overnight and drained
¾ cup (180 milliliters) Clearly Coconut Water (page 145) or bottled raw
  coconut water
⅔ cup (100 grams) maple sugar
½ teaspoon ground cinnamon
½ teaspoon vanilla powder (see Note, page 162)
¼ teaspoon salt

[295]

In a blender, combine all the ingredients and blend from low to high speed until silky smooth, stopping to scrape the sides of the machine once or twice. Transfer to a container, cover, and refrigerate for a couple of hours to firm up, then spoon into dessert bowls and serve.

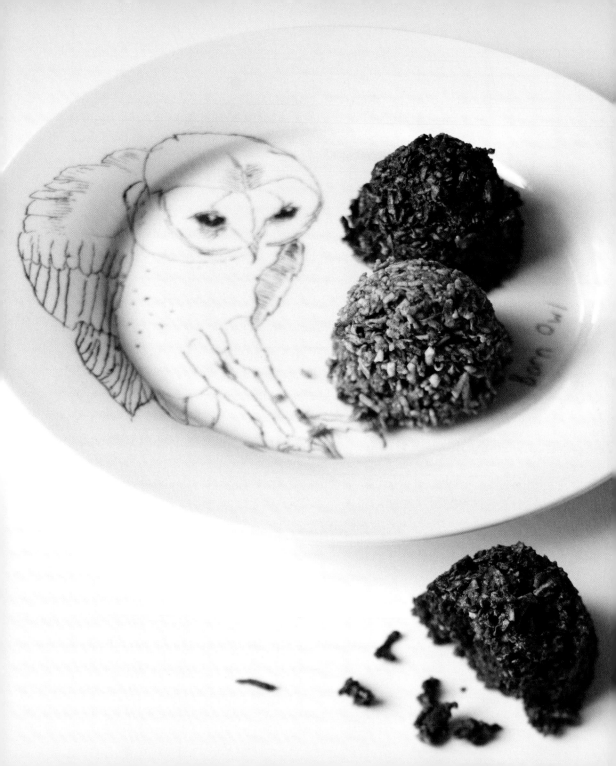

Choice Chocolate Macaroons

Sweetened with coconut sugar and deeply flavored with chocolate, these macaroons are ones you'll linger over and make again and again. Though they require some time in the dehydrator, putting them together involves just about ten minutes of active prep time, a sweet reward indeed.

Makes about 2 dozen

3 cups (8 ounces/225 grams) unsweetened shredded coconut
1 cup (4 ounces/120 grams) coconut sugar
⅔ cup (2 ounces/45 grams) cocoa powder
2 teaspoons vanilla powder (see Note, page 162)
Small pinch of salt
½ cup (120 milliliters) melted coconut oil
½ cup (120 milliliters) water

In a large bowl, combine the coconut, coconut sugar, cocoa powder, vanilla powder, and salt. Add the coconut oil and water and work the liquid ingredients in with your hands until they are incorporated and the texture resembles wet sand. Make sure the ingredients are thoroughly mixed with the liquid to avoid clumping.

[297]

Using a 1-ounce cookie scoop, scoop the mixture onto two ParaFlexx-lined dehydrator sheets. Set the machine to 110°F (40°C) and dehydrate for 5 hours, or until slightly firm on the outside and soft on the inside. Store in a covered container for up to 2 weeks.

Snazzy Snickerdoodle Macaroons

Based on the old-fashioned New England cinnamon-spiked cookie of the same name, our version becomes a snickerdoodle-macaroon hybrid gone vegan, done so with a triple treatment of coconut—shredded coconut, coconut sugar, and coconut oil—to complete the collaboration. Must be tasted to be believed!

Makes about 2 dozen

3 cups (8 ounces/225 grams) unsweetened shredded coconut
1 cup (4 ounces/120 grams) coconut sugar
½ cup (2 ounces/70 grams) lucuma powder
1 tablespoon vanilla powder (see Note, page 162)
1½ teaspoons ground cinnamon
¾ teaspoon freshly grated nutmeg
Small pinch of ground cloves
Small pinch of salt
½ cup (120 milliliters) melted coconut oil
½ cup (120 milliliters) water

In a large bowl, combine the coconut, coconut sugar, lucuma powder, vanilla powder, cinnamon, nutmeg, cloves, and salt. Add the coconut oil and water and work the liquid ingredients in with your hands until they are incorporated and the texture resembles wet sand. Make sure the ingredients are thoroughly mixed with the liquid to avoid clumping.

Using a 1-ounce cookie scoop, scoop the mixture onto two ParaFlexx-lined dehydrator sheets. Set the machine to 110°F (40°C) and dehydrate for 5 hours, or until slightly firm on the outside and soft on the inside. Store in a covered container for up to 2 weeks.

LIVING FOODS: IT'S REALLY NOTHING NEW
It's actually a concept borrowed from ancient civilizations! The Essenes, a Jewish sect dating from before the time of Jesus, were said to eat primarily live foods and were reported by anthropological historians to live an average of 120 years.

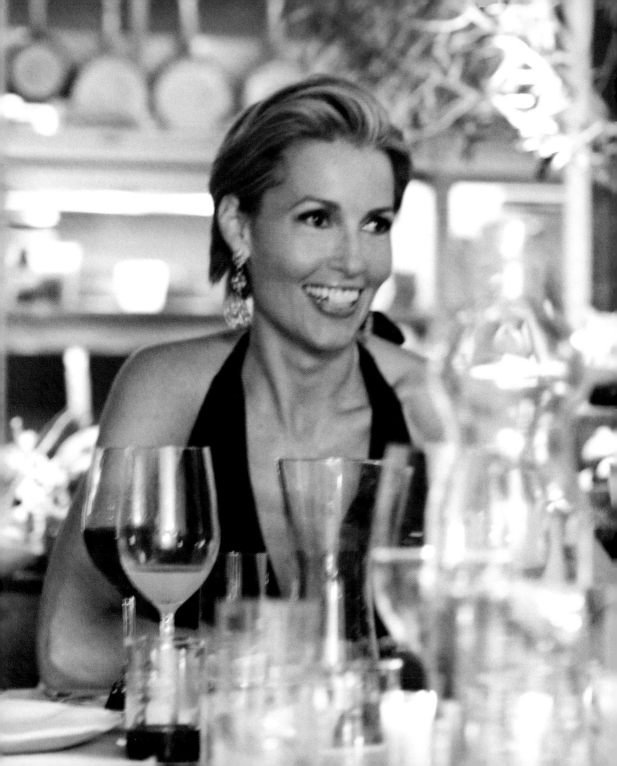

PART V

Bringing the LOVE* Home: Final Musings on the Live. Organic. Vegan. Experience.

Life is about connection. And meaningful connection often takes place over great food. Actually, almost everything takes place over food. Whether it is a traditional celebration, holiday, family gathering, or date, you will find that food is almost always at the center. And partaking in gatherings around LOVE*Food is an incredible way to increase a spiritual focus in life. Now as much as I LOVE* this concept, the reality is that it's a slim (no pun intended) few who get to indulge in LOVE*Food *and* family connection time. It is not always easy to bring this conversation home (unless that is where it started). This is why it is important to find a community of friends who support your transition toward healthful, life-affirming foods and practices.

> **Find your group: A nonjudgmental and awakened group of people who support a cleansing vegan lifestyle is the best form of support."**
> —DENISE MARI

Of course, in the real world, it is not easy to find a community that embraces this. Instead, you must "be the change" you wish to see in the world (in Gandhi's terms). That is where the magic is. It's not in telling others what they should and shouldn't do. It's developing the dedication to living life fully, which means loving your family, participating in celebrations, feeling good in your heart, being you, and letting go of what others are doing and expecting. We all change, grow, and evolve at our own pace and to the extent of our desire. We cannot force others to join us on our journey, no matter how much we think we know what is best for those around us.

> **Love is the strongest force the world possesses, and yet it is the humblest imaginable."**
> —MAHATMA GANDHI

Yet when you know what you are choosing is best for not only you, but also the animals and planet—the whole of us all—you know you are right where you are supposed to be. Yes, the contrast between you and those who are not living a LOVE*ing life will increase as you become witness to a growing peace within while continuing to be present to the vast amount of pain and suffering around you. Keep faith that with the persistent positive intention that you bring to your meals (yes, your meals) and your lifestyle choices, you will evolve and attract new energy. It may be energy that shows you who or what you are to become, it may be a light that continues to guide your path with a faint whisper that will get louder the longer you commit. Sitting still, being at peace, being in acceptance of friends, family, and loved ones, and being your new self along the way is all part of the equation that makes this world the beautiful place it is.

So on a practical level, how do you maintain this good vibe you picked up during your cleansing process? How can you keep it flowing so you can continue to thrive on inspiration and love your body the whole way through? Guess what? It's simple! There is a learning curve, but it generally comes down to the consciousness you bring to each situation. I hope you will enjoy the LOVE*Food recipes I've provided and that they inspire you to further develop your kitchen skills. Raw food can be a way of life; I was eating all raw foods for five years, and those were some of the best years of my life. But sometimes staying "all raw" is not an option. I myself now choose to eat some comforting cooked foods from time to time (between cleanses), and I find it to be a nice middle ground. It's not an all-or-nothing game. It's about having the tools for healing, boosting your nutritional intake, allowing your body to cleanse healthfully, and then also being a part of the real world—the one we live in. We are not all going to run off to the mountains and meditate; we can meditate from home and find our way right here by choosing a plant-based diet to keep our consciousness and bodies alive.

In metropolitan areas like New York City, we are blessed—the vegan movement is well under way and there is no shortage of everything from casual to fine dining, from pure raw to straight vegan, vegan Japanese, Korean, Italian, and Chinese. If you are traveling, do what I do: Take a look at the happycow .net site or other foodie sites that give you the lowdown on the vegan action in the area you are visiting. Enjoy dining at vegan and vegan-friendly restaurants. Look online for local farmers' markets, natural food stores, and juice bars as well. Go to your favorite restaurant or try a new one. Be the first to request vegan food, and I promise you won't be the last; you just may make it easier on the next person. It's always good to call ahead if you can; this way the chef has time to prepare and be even more thoughtful. Over the years (and it's taken years) I've learned to scan the menu quickly and see what vegetables and fruits they are serving, then use the menu as an ingredient list to see if I can create my own salad, or find the most veg-heavy item on the menu and have them remove anything non-veg. There is so much satisfaction from eating well when

[303]

traveling. There is so much joy in taking care of oneself no matter what the challenge.

When it comes to family gatherings, do your best. Offer to bring a dish, eat before you go, respond lovingly to questions but change the subject if you feel the conversation becoming hostile (remember your goals of being the change and shining bright lights on a room that not all are ready to see). Believe me, I know how hard it can be. Stay humble and helpful, and turn the conversation in the direction of loving goodness. It's all a practice. And as time goes on, you will become masterful at it.

And when you're feeling overwhelmed, simply remember that a healthy vegan diet is one based on eating plants, and to look for the number 9 on the PLU of your produce, which indicates that it was organically grown. And if that number 9 is driving you a little nutty, go straight to your local organic farmer. Or better yet, start a garden and grow your own: Talk about self-reliance and empowerment! If those options are not ringing as answers to your organic produce needs, consider a CSA (community supported agriculture) program, where you buy advance shares in a farm's growing season and reap the rewards throughout the season, or if you're a real convenience junkie, move close to an Organic Avenue and we'll take care of everything for you (online programs are available too—we'll do anything to support your path toward LOVE*!).

Finally, what I find most essential is knowing *why* you are choosing the LOVE*Lifestyle. Become educated in all things vegan, raw, and organic. Learn about the truth involving your food and your choices. Search the PETA (People for the Ethical Treatment of Animals) website. Discover the reality behind the animal industry; visit a slaughterhouse. Watch *Earthlings,* a documentary on the suffering of animals; *Fast Food Nation,* an exposé of the fast-food industry; or *Forks over Knives,* a movie about the link between animal-based foods and disease. Read or listen to an audio download of T. Colin Campbell's *China Study* (I listened to it multiple times), one of the strongest cases for veganism to date; study alkalinity from the perspective of *The pH Miracle* author Dr. Robert O.

[304]

Young—see what you think and then test it all for yourself. Learn how to get your voice heard and demand that GMOs be labeled (better yet, just say no! no! no!). Follow doctors favoring plant-based diets like Dr. John McDougall, Dr. Caldwell Esselstyn, and Dr. Colin Campbell. Be thrilled by the athletes who are raw and vegan. Log on to the truthabouthealth.org website, attend retreats at a place like the Ann Wigmore Institute in Puerto Rico or Optimum Health Institute or We Care Spa in California (see Resources, page 307). Connect to the experience of people who have been living the lifestyle for many years, and trust that this is a possibility for you, too!

The movement toward truth, health, and environment is well under way. Join the network and find your own way of linking your passion, truth, and voice to a greater cause. Know why you are making the choices you are making: from a nutritional perspective, from a compassionate perspective, from an environmental and even spiritual perspective. There is no shortage of good reasons to pursue LOVE*. And when you are armed with the knowledge and tools to live healthfully and happily, it makes it all that much easier to stay connected to this gateway into a better life. Knowledge is king, and experience queen: Together they make the perfect couple. And remember, just do it for the LOVE* of it!

[305]

Truly,
Denise Mari

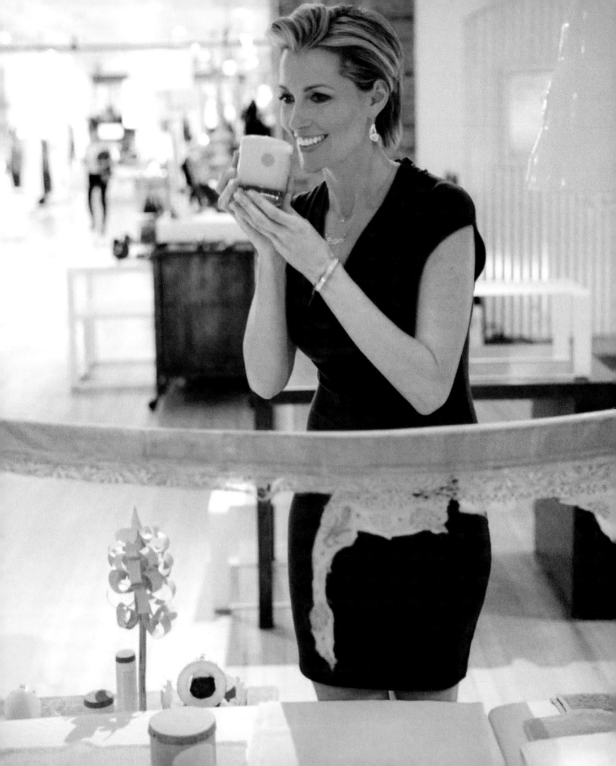

Resources: Finding the LOVE* All Around You

Denise Mari
For all things LOVE*
www.DeniseMari.com
Blog, events, product reviews, action links, recipes, support, and access to Mari Manor, a cleanse/detox retreat center in Westhampton Beach, New York

Online Cleanses
Organic Avenue
www.OrganicAvenue.com
Organic and vegan retail and home delivery of raw and consciously cooked food, juice, cleanse packages, and support

Health Experts and Recommended Books
Dr. Neal Barnard
www.nealbarnard.org
Health and nutrition advocate; author of *Power Foods for the Brain*

Victoria, Sergei, and Valya Boutenko
(aka The Raw Family)
www.rawfamily.com
Green smoothie and raw food experts; authors of *Green for Life* and *Green Smoothie Revolution*

Dr. T. Colin Campbell
www.tcolincampbell.org
Author of *The China Study*

Dr. David Carmos and Dr. Shawn Miller
Essene scholars; authors of *You're Never Too Old to Become Young*

Kris Carr
www.kriscarr.com
Wellness activist and cancer thriver; author of *Crazy Sexy Kitchen*

Gabriel Cousens
www.gabrielcousens.com
Live-food medical doctor and
detoxification expert; author of *Conscious
Eating* and *Rainbow Green Live-Food
Cuisine*

Dr. Caldwell B. Esselstyn
www.heartattackproof.com
Nutrition-oriented M.D.; author of
Prevent and Reverse Heart Disease

Doug Evans
www.dougevans.com
doug@dougevans.com
Raw vegan entrepreneur, life coach,
mentor, and conscious investor

Dr. Richard Firshein
www.firsheincenter.com
Founder and director of The Firshein
Center for Comprehensive Medicine
in New York City; author of *The
Neutraceutical Revolution*

Kathy Freston
www.kathyfreston.com
Healthy living and conscious eating
writer; author of *Veganist*

Dr. Joel Fuhrman
www.drfuhrman.com
Nutritional medicine M.D.; author of *Eat
to Live*

Dr. Oz Garcia
www.ozgarcia.com
Leading authority on healthy aging
and nutritionist to the stars; author of
Redesigning 50

Dr. Max Gerson
www.gerson.org
Founder of the Gerson Therapy, a whole-
body approach to healing emphasizing
fresh juices; author of *A Cancer Therapy*

Dr. Douglas Graham
www.foodnsport.com
Raw food athlete; author of *Nutrition and
Athletic Performance*

Dr. Bernard Jensen
Proponent of iridology, colon
hydrotherapy, and other alternative
cure methods; author of many books,
including *Dr. Jensen's Guide to Better
Bowel Care*

Dr. Alejandro Junger
www.cleanprogram.com
Cardiologist and cleanse specialist;
author of *Clean Gut*

Ashley Koff, RD
www.ashleykoffapproved.com
Qualitarian, nutrition expert, and speaker;
author of *Mom Energy*

Dr. John A. McDougall
www.drmcdougall.com
Diet and lifestyle medicine specialist;
author of *The McDougall Program*

Gary Null
www.thegarynullshow.podbean.com
Alternative and complementary medicine
expert and nutrition talk show host;
author of *The Complete Encyclopedia of
Natural Healing*

Dr. Dean Ornish
www.ornishspectrum.com
The first to connect lifestyle changes
with reversing heart disease; author of
*Dr. Dean Ornish's Program for Reversing
Heart Disease*

Karen Ranzi
www.superhealthychildren.com
Nutrition and child development expert;
author of *Creating Healthy Children*

John Robbins
www.johnrobbins.com
Spokesman for an ethical and sustainable
future; author of *Diet for a New America*
and *The Food Revolution*

Natalia Rose
www.detoxtheworld.com
Clinical nutritionist and cleanse expert

Alicia Silverstone
www.thekindlife.com
Animal rights and environmental activist;
author of *The Kind Diet*

Norman W. Walker
Vegetable juicing pioneer; author of *Colon
Health: The Key to a Vibrant Life*

Ann Wigmore
www.wigmore.org
Whole foods advocate and wheatgrass
guru; author of *The Wheatgrass Book* and
The Hippocrates Diet and Health Program

David Wolfe
www.davidwolfe.com
Superfood and longevity expert; author
of *The Sunfood Diet Success System* and
*Superfoods: The Food and Medicine of
the Future*

Dr. Robert O. Young
www.phmiracleliving.com
Alkaline diet expert; author of *The pH
Miracle*

[309]

Some Favorite Cookbooks

Carol Alt, *Easy Sexy Raw: 130 Raw Food Recipes, Tools, and Tips to Make You Feel Gorgeous and Satisfied* (Clarkson Potter, 2012); *Eating in the Raw: A Beginner's Guide to Getting Slimmer, Feeling Healthier, and Looking Younger the Raw-Food Way* (Clarkson Potter, 2004)

Matt Amsden, *RAWvolution: Gourmet Living Cuisine* (William Morrow, 2006)

Karyn Calabrese, *Soak Your Nuts: Karyn's Conscious Comfort Foods* (Book Publishing Co., 2013)

Terces Engelhart, *I Am Grateful: Recipes and Lifestyle of Café Gratitude* (North Atlantic Books, 2007)

Kathy Freston, *Veganist: Lose Weight, Get Healthy, Change the World* (Weinstein Books, 2011)

Juliano, *Raw: The Uncook Book* (Regan Books, 1999)

Matthew Kenney, *Everyday Raw Gourmet* (Gibbs Smith, 2013) and many other cookbooks

Leslie McEachern, *The Angelica Home Kitchen: Recipes and Rabble Rousings from an Organic Vegan Restaurant* (Ten Speed Press, 2003)

Sarma Melngailis, *Living Raw Food: Get the Glow with More Recipes from Pure Food and Wine* (William Morrow, 2009); *Raw Food/Real World: 100 Recipes to Get the Glow* (William Morrow, 2005)

Erin Pavlina, *Vegan Family Favorites: Tasty and Satisfying Recipes Even Your Kids Will Love* (VegFamily, 2006); *Raising Vegan Children in a Non-Vegan World: A Complete Guide for Parents* (VegFamily, 2003)

Tanya Petrovna, *The Native Foods Restaurant Cookbook: Fresh, Fun, and Delicious Vegan Recipes That Will Entice and Satisfy Vegetarians and Nonvegetarians Alike* (Shambhala, 2003)

Ani Phyo, *Ani's Raw Food Essentials: Recipes and Techniques for Mastering the Art of Live Food* (Da Capo, 2010); *Ani's Raw Food Desserts: 85 Easy, Delectable Sweets and Treats* (Da Capo, 2009); *Ani's Raw Food Kitchen: Easy, Delectable Living Foods Recipes* (Da Capo, 2007)

Joy Pierson and Bart Potenza, *The Candle Café Cookbook: More Than 150 Enlightened Recipes from New York's Renowned Vegan Restaurant* (Clarkson Potter, 2003)

Rhio: *Hooked on Raw: Rejuvenate Your Body and Soul with Nature's Living Foods* (Book Publishing Co., 2000)

Matthew Rogers, Tiziana Alipo Tamborra, and Terces Engelhart, *Sweet Gratitude: A New World of Raw Desserts* (North Atlantic Books, 2008)

Herbert M. Shelton, *Food Combining Made Easy* (Book Publishing Co., 2012)

Cheryl Stoycoff, *Raw Kids: Transitioning Children to a Raw Food Diet* (Living Spirit Press, 2004)

Renée Loux Underkoffler, *Living Cuisine: The Art and Spirit of Raw Foods* (Avery, 2004)

Tonya Zavasta, *Your Right to Be Beautiful: The Miracle of Raw Foods* (BR Publishing, 2003)

Movies to Mull Over

Babe (1995)

The Beautiful Truth (2008)

Charlotte's Web (1973)

The Cove (2009)

A Cow at My Table (1998)

Dying to Have Known (2006)

Earthlings (2005)

Fast Food Nation (2006)

Fat, Sick, and Nearly Dead (2010)

Food, Inc. (2008)

Food Matters (2008)

Forks over Knives (2011)

The Future of Food (2004)

Got the Facts on Milk? The Milk Documentary (2011)

May I Be Frank (2010)

No Impact Man (2009)

Raw for Life/Simply Raw (2011)

A Sacred Duty: Applying Jewish Values to Help Heal the World (2007)

Simply Raw: Reversing Diabetes in 30 Days (2009)

Super Size Me (2004)

Vegucated (2010)

The World According to Monsanto (2008)

Educational Programs of Interest

Ann Wigmore Natural Health Institute

www.annwigmore.org

787-504-1329

Living Foods Lifestyle Certification Program in Puerto Rico

eCornell Certificate in Plant-Based Nutrition

www.ecornell.com/I-PBN

866-326-7635

Three-course series with Dr. T. Colin Campbell

[311]

Hippocrates Health Institute
www.hippocratesinst.org/the-institute
561-471-8876
Life Transformation Program and Health
Educator Program in southern Florida

Institute for Integrative Nutrition
www.integrativenutrition.com
877-730-5444
Health coach training program in New
York City

Living Light Culinary Institute
Raw vegan chef training program in
California
www.rawfoodchef.com
800-816-2319

Matthew Kenney Academy
www.matthewkenneycuisine.com/
education
Raw and living foods educational center
in Santa Monica and Miami

Pure Joy Academy
www.purejoyacademy.com
Raw food chef and health educator
certification course in Los Angeles and
Sedona

Raw Chef Dan
www.rawchefdan.com
Raw Foods A to Z Certification Training in
New York City

Websites

Chic Vegan
www.chicvegan.com
Vegan lifestyle site

Choose Veg
www.chooseveg.com
Vegan recipes and lifestyle tips

Crazy Sexy Wellness
www.kriscarr.com
Site of Kris Carr, wellness activist and
cancer thriver

Girlie Girl Army
www.girliegirlarmy.com
Vegan guide to conscious living

Happy Cow
HappyCow.net
Healthy eating guide for when you're out
and about

The Kind Life
www.thekindlife.com
Alicia Silverstone's vegan website

MindBodyGreen
www.mindbodygreen.com
Website dedicated to making wellness
fun and inclusive

PETA (People for the Ethical Treatment of Animals)
PETA.org
World's largest animal rights organization

Physicians Committee for Responsible Medicine
www.pcrm.org
Promotion of preventive medicine

SuperVegan
Blog and New York City Vegan restaurant guide
www.supervegan.com

Vegan Bodybuilding & Fitness
Vegan training and fitness
www.veganbodybuilding.com

VegGuide
Vegetarian and Vegan restaurant guide
www.vegguide.org

Well + Good
Health, beauty, and fitness site
www.wellandgoodnyc.com

LOVE*-Friendly Retreats: Vacations for Health

Amansala
www.amansalaresort.com
Eco-chic resort and spa in Mexico

Ann Wigmore Institute
www.annwigmore.org
787-868-6307
Puerto Rico oceanside retreat based on Dr. Ann Wigmore's Living Food Lifestyle

David Wolfe Adventures
www.davidwolfeadventures.com
Worldwide trips designed to nourish the health and soul

Dr. Cousens' Tree of Life Rejuvenation Center
www.treeoflife.nu
866-394-2520
Holistic lifestyle campus, vegan healing center, and spiritual community in Arizona

Garden Diet
www.28daysraw.com
Twenty-eight day online raw foods transition program

Grace Grove Lifestyle Center
www.gracegrove.com
Detoxification and rejuvenation retreats in Arizona

[313]

Hippocrates Health Institute
www.hippocratesinst.org
888-228-1755
Florida-based complementary health-
care center founded by Ann Wigmore and
directed by Dr. Brian Clement and Dr.
Anna Maria Clement

Mari Manor
www.MariManor.com
An ahimsa-conscious organic, vegan
retreat center, bed and breakfast, and
bed and cleanse located in Westhampton
Beach, Long Island, New York

Optimum Health Institute
www.optimumhealth.org
800-993-4325
Body, mind, spirit program in Texas

**ph Miracle Private Retreats at Rancho
Del Sol**
www.phmiracleliving.com
760-751-8321
Dr. Robert D. Young's lifestyle and dietary
program

The Ranch
www.theranchmalibu.com
888-777-2177
Fitness and wellness immersion in
California

We Care
www.wecarespa.com
800-888-2523
Juice fasting spiritual retreat in California

Sustainable Home Furnishings

ABC Carpet & Home
www.abchome.com
Large and varied home furnishing
selection, textiles, tabletops, clothing,
and beauty products (products featured
in cover shot, all recipe shots, and
pages x, 123, 192, 300, and 306)

Gaiam
www.gaiam.com
Sustainable furniture and lifestyle
products

Compassionate Clothing

Alternative Outfitters
www.alternativeoutfitters.com
Vegan boutique

Beyond Skin
www.beyondskin.co.uk
Vegan footwear

Bourgeois Boheme
www.bboheme.com
Vegan footwear

Compassion Couture
www.compassioncoutureshop.com
Cruelty-free and eco-friendly boutique

Cow Jones Industrials
www.cowjonesindustrials.com
Vegan clothing boutique

Ethical Ocean
www.ethicalocean.com
All things eco

Faerie's Dance
www.faeriesdance.com
Earth-friendly fashions

The Hempest
www.store.hempest.com
Hemp clothing

The Herbivore Clothing Company
www.herbivoreclothing.com
Eco clothing

Kaight
www.kaightshop.com
Eco fashions

Loomstate
www.loomstate.org
Socially and environmentally friendly
fashion

Matt & Nat
www.mattandnat.com
Large selection of nonleather bags

Moo Shoes
www.mooshoes.com
Vegan footwear and accessories

Rapanui
www.rapanuiclothing.com
Eco fashion

Rogan R44
www.r44roganstandardissue.tumblr.com
Organic clothing line

Stella McCartney
www.stellamccartney.com
Designer clothing with social awareness

Vaute Couture
www.vautecouture.com
Vegan clothing line

[315]

Cosmetics

Cruelty-Free Face
www.crueltyfreeface.com
Educational site on compassionate
cosmetics

Marie Veronique Organics
www.mvorganics.com
Intelligent, sustainable ingredients

Obsessive Compulsive Cosmetics
www.occmakeup.com
Vegan and cruelty-free cosmetics

Food and Equipment Sources

Comprehensive Food and Equipment Sites

High Vibe
www.highvibe.com
888-554-6645
Large selection of live foods, superfoods, supplements, and appliances

Live Live & Organic
www.live-live.com
877-505-5504
Many LOVE* basics, including dehydrators, juicers, nut milk bags, spiral slicers, sprouters, books, DVDs, green powders, kelp noodles, seaweeds, sweeteners, and other foods

Longevity Warehouse
www.longevitywarehouse.com
805-870-5756

Large selection of superfoods; spirulina, chlorella, mesquite, lucuma, seaweeds, cacao powder, goji berries, coconut oil, and other foods

Raw Food World Store
www.therawfoodworld.com
866-729-3438
Many LOVE* basics, including dehydrators, juicers, nut milk bags, spiral slicers, sprouters, books, DVDs, chlorella, E3, spirulina, and other supplements, Irish moss, nuts, seeds, seaweed products, protein powder, sweeteners, and other foods

Specialized Food Product Sites

Coconut Secret
www.coconutsecret.com
888-369-3393
Coconut sugar

Divine Organics
www.divineorganics.com
415-884-4477
Raw coconut blossom sugar (creamy coconut sugar), coconut water, frozen coconut meat

Sea Tangle Noodle Company
www.kelpnoodles.com
408-966-3109
Kelp noodles

Supplements

Bōku
www.bokusuperfood.com
877-265-8366
Protein powder and superfood supplements, matcha green tea powder

E3 Live
www.e3live.com
888-800-7070
Blue-green algae

Innate Response Formulas
www.innateresponse.com
800-634-6342
Whole food–passed supplements

Mega Food
www.megafood.com
High-quality supplements

pHMiracleLiving
www.pHmiracleliving.com
760-751-8321
Alkalizing water machines, cleansing supplements including pH drops

Vitamin Code
www.thevitamincode.com
Raw food–based nutrients

[318]

Juicers

Breville
www.brevilleusa.com
Centrifugal juicer

Champion
www.championjuicer.com
866-935-8423
Masticating juicer

Green Star
www.greenstar.com
888-254-7336
Twin-gear press juicer

Jack La Lanne's Power Juicer
www.powerjuicer.com
Centrifugal juicer

Juicero
www.juicero.com
917-859-7384
info@juicero.com
Cold-press juicing systems

Norwalk
www.norwalkjuicers.com
800-643-8645
Grind and press juicer

Nutri Bullet
www.nutribullet.com
800-370-0653
Superfood Nutrition Extractor

Dehydrators

Excalibur
www.excaliburdehydrator.com
800-875-4254
Multishelf dehydrators

Blenders

Blendtec
www.blendtec.com
801-222-0888
High-speed blender

Vitamix
www.vitamix.com
800-848-2649
High-speed blender

[319]

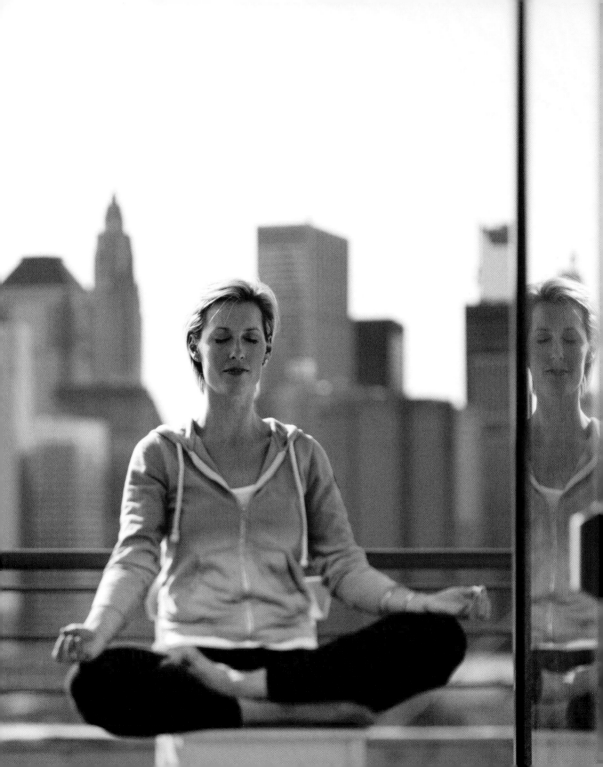

Acknowledgments

With Gratitude

Thank you, Lisa Sharkey, for recognizing the LOVE* and taking it all to the next level! Perfect timing! I knew from the start I would be in good hands with you and HarperCollins. Through your guidance, support, and faith in me and Organic Avenue, this book (G-d willing) will reach many readers and lives will be spared and improved. Special thanks to Amy Bendell for all your hard work and support and to the HarperCollins team for being believers early on and for giving me a platform to share.

Leda Scheintaub, you are an angel of patience and perseverance. Thank you for pouring your love into every page of this book and going above and beyond the call of duty. Knowing each recipe was tested to perfection assures me that the reader is getting an authentic LOVE* Lifestyle experience as they re-create these recipes at home. Thank you from the bottom of my heart. There would be no book of LOVE* without you.

Debra Winter, angels come at perfect times; when needed most, they appear. Your guiding love came in perfect time to ease the transition and prepare for new life to come. Words don't do justice to the feeling of gratitude I have for your encouragement, patience, creative support, and all the hours you labored over this book with love.

Thank you, Paulette Cole, CEO of ABC Carpet & Home, for your unwavering support of Organic Avenue, and for lending your creative vision and direction along with your wonderful team: Amy Chender and Amy Alias. Thank you for supporting and encouraging my passion in the early days when Organic Avenue was a budding home-based business, and for working on this book as if it were your own! I'm honored to have had such an all-star team giving last-minute love against all odds and accommodating with grace and kindness (even during the busiest season)! The artistic intention shines through each and every photo. I'm deeply grateful.

Quentin Bacon, thank you for making the book come to life with your brilliant photographs and for capturing the glamorous aspect of the vegan lifestyle. You are a true pleasure to work with!

Organic Avenue team members, past and present, you supported a dream and it became a reality. You've contributed to the growth of more than a retail chain; you've given life to a dream that is changing lives, saving innocent beings, and protecting our planet. Thank you all!

Stephen Mahabir, thank you for helping in the kitchen as we were compiling the recipes for this book. Mercedes Anna Martinez, you are an angel for lending your creative chef talent to the process. It was wonderful working with you!

Jonathan Grayer, every angel has his form. Thank you!

Martin Bates, I am grateful for your contribution and your shown ability to grasp the magnitude of the Vision and to guide Organic Avenue to its most beautiful expression.

The early believers: Joel Schrieber, Eric Cahan, Joel Seiden, Laurin Seiden, Evan Seiden, the Niven Family, Arthur Pergament and family, Paulette Cole, Josh Mailman, John and Michael Warburg, Joe Ferreira, Greg Brenner, Rita Thomas, John Edelman.

Howard Kesseler, I am grateful for our inspired connection. I believe in miracles!

The one and only Doug Evans! A floating chance meeting that led to the greatest Light. Thank you for your inspired teachings and freedom to fly. You are a tremendous example of what *to* do. I leapt because you did! And for believing in the vision from its smallest seed to its global intention and for staying by my side through the adventure. Your boundless enthusiasm, entrepreneurial genius, and loyal friendship have shaped Organic Avenue into what it is today! It's been an amazing ride. What's next?!

My family: Kimberly, your innocent life lost gave mine meaningful direction. You have not been forgotten. Michele, for teaching me about my nature and being my loving little sister. John, for being a creative big brother (you led the way into trouble . . . and then I took over from there); for finding your spiritual connection and keeping it real for your family. Mom, example of selflessness, unconditional love, and enduring patience—I miss you. Dad, for giving your all to our family. You did good! And to Kylee, Aiden, Suzanne, and Kimberly for bringing new light and life to our family. I love you all!

Oliver, my son, moon, and stars. Thank you for being so I could love more deeply. I love you. Always.

Great One, Mother, Father, Light, Divine Force, the Nameless One, I bow my head to thee in reverence for your divine presence and teachings. May I walk with you always, in my heart, in my soul, trusting your will for me. With a soul full of gratitude, I give thanks.

[323]

Special Thanks

To those who have contributed, supported, inspired, touched, shaped, influenced, or loved me to be who I am, and therefore brought this book into being:

David Wolfe, a leading example of fearlessness and forgiveness, passion and purpose, for pioneering a movement toward the truth in nutrition and for leading in creativity and enthusiasm, from the early days at Eden Hot Springs to the Longevity conferences of today. We need only to look to you to find the most cutting-edge information on nutrition science and superfoods. Grow, NoniLand, grow!

Jill Pettijohn, for your sisterhood, inspiration, and support in taking the first juice-cleanse experience from the loft days of Organic Avenue on the Lower East Side and guiding OA's launch onto the streets of New York City.

Dr. Shawn Miller, for living the path less chosen and for finding the deeper meaning in it all. Thank you for sharing the LOVE* (literally and figuratively)! It's made its mark on the world. The ripple effect has begun.

Dr. Robert O. Young, for your inspiring life's work and mission.

David Ghiyam, for bringing new Light to my life and keeping it shining.

Frank Anguili, for trusting me with a bag of Natural High Lifestyle hemp/organic clothing to sell at a retreat and launching me and Organic Avenue into business.

Jamie Richardson, for being my first-ever vegetarian friend.

Matt Stone and the Allegro Team, and Gidon, for the behind-the-scenes essential tech wizardry.

Joshua Rosenthal, for teaching open-minded health and nutrition practices and entrepreneurship, freeing many to serve in truly meaningful ways.

Others who have inspired, directed, taught, and led the way by their example and their steadfast determination to be, practice, and stand for the truth: the Boutenko family, Dr. David Carmos, Dr. Brian Clement, and Dr. Gabriel Cousens.

Special chefs who have influenced the ever-delicious diversity of Organic Avenue's menu: Michele Thorne, Scott Winegard, Matteo Silverman, Pete Cervoni, Mercedes Anna Martinez, and Magnus Hansson; Elaina Love, Mathew Kenney, Sarma Melngailis, Juliano, Renee Loux, Jeremy Saffron, Matt Samuelson, Chad Sarno, Dan Hoyt, and Tolentin Chan.

Loving friends and contributors not to be forgotten for their unconditional support and enthusiasm for the mission and me: Lisa Paris, Jenna Preuss, Richard Rubenstein, Nancy Trent, Kari Neering, Paul Hwang, Colin Beavan, David Feece, Ryan Harbage, Sisters of Eden, Lynley Swain, Giselle Tarres, Kim Sol, Anahata, Puma, Paola Guillen, Karen Clement, Natane Boudreau, and Cole Lopez.

The Weld North Team, for giving all things LOVE* and Organic Avenue the wings to fly and the support to stay afloat! Remember: **Do it for the LOVE* of it!**

[324]

Credits

Denise Mari: Organic Avenue founder, author, and creative director

Leda Scheintaub: writer, recipe development and testing

Debra Winter: contributing writer, creative contributions, project manager

Quentin Bacon: photography; Kristen Walther, assistant

ABC Carpet & Home: creative direction, prop sourcing

Mariana Velasquez: food styling

Suzanne Lenzer: prop and food styling

Maeve Sheridan: prop styling

Wilhelmina Talent: hair, makeup, styling

Mercedes Anna Martinez, Magnus Hansson, Pete Cervoni: chef and recipe
development

Baruch Gorkin: Organic Avenue corporate identity and design contributions

Anja Schutz: Organic Avenue original logo illustration

Index

[327]

[329]

[331]